EDWARD COTTER

Homoeopathic Teachings from a Master

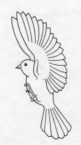

SAFFRON WALDEN
THE C.W. DANIEL COMPANY LIMITED

First published in Great Britain in 1987
by The C. W. Daniel Company Limited
1 Church Path, Saffron Walden, Essex, England

© Phyllis Speight 1987

ISBN 0 85207 183 3

Set in 10/11 point Souvenir by
MS Typesetting, Castle Camps, Cambridge and printed by
Hillman Printers (Frome) Ltd., Frome, Somerset, England

Contents

Introduction

The title of this book was carefully chosen and it was not, in any way, meant to be presumptuous.

But let me start at the beginning.

Edward Cotter was introduced to Leslie and me by one of our leading homoeopathic physicians.

It was a delight to both of us to get to know, and love a man who was reserved, who shunned publicity but who had a deep knowledge and love of classical Homoeopathy.

He had a large and thriving practice in the West End of London, his patients coming from all walks of life, including well-known names from politics, the stage and, yes doctors.

He was reluctant to associate with practitioners who did not understand and work according to the laws laid down by Samuel Hahnemann.

Edward became very interested in 'The Homoeopathic World' which, at that time, we had revived and we were delighted when he was persuaded to contribute articles. These are presented here in book form in Edward's clear and precise manner, which to me, is a reflection of his uncluttered mind.

For the keen student there is help to understand case taking and information about repertorising which is a very misunderstood aspect of homoeopathy.

For others there are directions for the use of common remedies for every day injuries and mishaps, and the numerous case histories demonstrate how Homoeopathy can deal with troubles that are often considered incurable by other means.

This book will be very helpful to students who wish to learn classical Homoeopathy as taught by Hahnemann — there is a lesson in each article.

I still miss Edward very much, but am grateful for his friendship and help throughout the years until his death. He always had the answers to my problems but we laughed a lot too, for he had a great sense of humour.

Phyllis Speight

CHAPTER 1

What Homoeopathy Is and Is Not

1. HOMOEOPATHY is not new. Hippocrates, Galen, Holler, Stork and many other great teachers in medicine, were familiar with the homoeopathic law of cure, but it was not until over 150 years ago that Dr. Samuel Hahnemann (physician and scientist) first recognised its full value and made its application general.

2. HOMOEOPATHY stands on the solid rock of fact, unlike the succession of drugs constantly hailed as wonderful advances only to drop out of sight, if not memory, in a short time, only too often leaving behind a trail of human misery as a legacy of their brief existence. Homoeopathy has been tested daily for more than a century and a half and appreciation of its beneficient results by intelligent people in every community is stronger today than ever before.

3. HOMOEOPATHY is not a complicated proposition beyond the comprehension of thinking people. It rests upon a simple, demonstrable law of nature that pure medicine in small and gentle doses, accurately selected to fit the patient's requirements, will set that patient on the road to recovery.

4. HOMOEOPATHY is not guesswork nor a fine spun theory. Each one of the hundreds of medicines employed by homoeopaths has been proved or tested upon the healthy human organism, showing what organs, functions or structures it affects. Mark that these experiments were not made upon cats, dogs or guinea pigs, but upon hundreds of earnest men and women volunteers, who subjected themselves to pain and inconvenience for the purpose of helping the sick. This has given us absolute knowledge of our medicines and their curative virtues.

5. HOMOEOPATHY does not seek to palliate or to suppress pain. It goes to the *root of the trouble*, and for that very reason will overcome pain when drugs and other palliatives afford only temporary relief.

6. HOMOEOPATHY does not repress symptoms nor give temporary relief at the expense of future comfort and safety. It aims, by the remedy given, to reach the cause of the disturbance and thus make the sick well again.

7. HOMOEOPATHY does not and cannot injure the human system. Its effect is gentle. Its methods do not exhaust the patients vitality and therefore progress is not retarded. It instead coaxes back to health, and allows the carefully preserved vital energy to make recovery a rapid and safe process.

8. HOMOEOPATHY does not claim to be a universal panacea but in more than 150 years application in every part of the civilized world it has demonstrated its curative power in all known disease-conditions, at any time of life. It acts as promptly in the vigorous man and woman as in childhood. It does not take the place of the surgeon's knife but, when skilfully used, often does away with the necessity of operating.

CHAPTER 2

The Organon, The Guide

No one should ever expect to practise the homoeopathic art of healing successfully, who is not well trained in the principles upon which it is founded, as these are set forth in that marvellous book, the Organon. The highest standard of therapeutic achievement is not too high for everyone. It requires faithful application of remedies according to principles and nothing more, for the results attained are developed by nature herself, within the organism.

Give the homoeopathic remedies according to the doctrines which govern sickness and cure, and receive the reward, as moving pictures resolve from one scene to another — pain disappearing, bloom appearing on the skin, roundness replacing emaciation, activity succeeding to helplessness, joy and reason assuming their rightful place — as each remedy enters into the life of the individual according to its affinity and in exemplification of the Law of Cure.

The Teachings of the Organon, well founded upon the basic rock of inexorable truth, are so far ahead of the time in which they were given that modern science is just beginning to catch up with and to confirm them.

When we look back over the history of Homoeopathy and its early successes at the hands of Hahnemann himself and of such pioneers as Hartman, Stapf, Boenninghausen, Hering and Lippe, and then find them repeated in more recent times by Dunham, Nash, E. A. Farrington, H. A. Allen and many others; when we realise that all these men were trained in the doctrines presented in the Organon, we cannot but recognise how important this Organon-study must be as a basis for the study of homoeopathic medicine. Its great principles can never grow useless and out of date, as they are founded on eternal truths which must ever have a place in our lives, a use in our practice. Its truths are real, positive, eternal and self-evident, based upon the tangible facts gleaned from the life-long observation and personal experiences of Hahnemann.

The Force Within

The Organon leads us beneath the surface of things, away from external appearances and results of disorder, into the very presence of actual causes where we may learn how the sick are to be observed in their expressions, their needs made known and supplied. Hahnemann elsewhere declares that disease-producing or morbific forces can derange man's vital force only by acting upon it in a dynamic manner; that is to say, that as vital force is dynamic it can be disturbed only by other forces of a dynamic nature.

The Normal Man

The vital force is exerted from the interior to the exterior of the organism, from within outward, from centre to circumference, from above downward, from the individual to the mind, and from mind to body. This is in keeping with the modern doctrine in biology that all processes of growth are from within outward. This is considered as the *law of direction*, which governs the operation of vital force in all its processes of life and growth; the flow outward into the outermost, from things that are in the interior. It is through our understanding of this principle that the interior states may be discerned upon the exteriors of the life.

The Abnormal Man

The teachings of the Organon is that every true disease first begins in the innermost expressions of vital force. It follows, that the process of cure must begin in things that are innermost and proceed to things that are outermost; starting in the vital, and proceeding to things of the mind, and lastly to things of the body. Every individual in health becomes known to us through our observation of those features and expressions which are strange, rare and peculiar; we could not know one person from another unless each had some peculiar and characteristic feature and expressions which others did not show. We observe sick people upon the same principle that we do in health, and thus learn to individualise each patient.

These strange, rare and peculiar symptoms reveal to us the true image of the patient. Upon the totality of these strange, rare and peculiar symptoms the Organon teaches us to base the homoeopathic prescription. *Only by these peculiar symptoms can we find the true similimum.* The remedy that will cure when this group of symptoms is found, be they ever so few in number, a big step forward has been made in the search for the most suitable remedy. The ability to determine these strange, rare and peculiar symptoms is the one thing which spells success in the homoeopathic art, and reveals the work of a master.

The Remedy

Since the homoeopathic prescription must be based upon the totality of the symptoms which reveal the patient, it follows that a *similar symptom-picture* must be present *in the provings of the remedy selected.* The law of Similia demands that we find a correspondence and likeness between the patient's picture and the picture of the remedy. This correspondence can never be found in the picture presented by the diagnosis only, but by those things which are strange, rare and peculiar, exceptions to the things of the diagnosis. *When the individuality of the remedy corresponds to the individuality of the patient, then, and only then, can it be homoeopathic to a given case.* Upon the correct application of this principle rests the peculiarity and the success of homoeopathic cures.

Homoeopathy, then, as laid down by the Organon, becomes a matter of close study of individuals, requiring us first to know the normal individual as revealed by the peculiar features pertaining to the personality. When this is known, we may observe the patient as an individual revealed by strange, rare and peculiar symptoms of sickness. When we observe the three individualities: the normal man, the abnormal man and the remedy, we have observed the foundations upon which a sound practice of Homoeopathy may be established.

CHAPTER 3

Your Body is Wearing Out

Nowadays most people are becoming interested, strangely interested, in health and disease, and all want to know why their health has suffered. Every doctor is asked by his patient: "Why has this come upon me?"

There are the usual plausible explanations, such as a cold, a chill, indigestion, physical or nervous overstrain, inadequate food, over-eating, hasty eating, overwork, and if none of these banal causes seem responsible then the trouble is declared to be due to the ubiquitous germ. As regards germs, possibly there are two different views. There is the view that every, or almost every, disease is due to a specific micro-organism; and there is the view that decomposition, disease, faulty living, produce the specific disease germs.

There is, however, another and most potent cause of diseases and disorders which is hardly ever mentioned. It is to be found in the fact that our bodies are wearing out. I have known a very large number of excellent doctors, both allopathic and homoeopathic, and surgeons, and the young doctors are usually keen and enthusiastic. They are eager to give such and such specific for every disease. They can tell you a lot about germ disease. They are ready to give the usual injections and even submit themselves to the standardized treatments, while the young surgeons are sometimes over-anxious to operate. But the old and very much more experienced medical men are usually rather sceptical as regards many so called scientific treatments and operations. They have had too many disappointments, and when they themselves are ill, they often smilingly decline professional help. Why? Because they are more or less aware that their bodies are wearing out or are worn out and cannot withstand the crushing impact of many modern drugs. When the orthodox doctor gives advice to a patient who is wearing out or worn out, he examines the individual and finds, let us say, some weakness in the heart or liver or arteries, for which he prescribes the standard or current treatment.

The homoeopath acts in rather a different manner. He notices, of course, that there is some weakness about some organ or organs for which he wishes to prescribe, and he also notices, as does his orthodox colleague, that the man's bodily machinery has run down rather badly. Being a homoeopath he does not give a 'specific' or current drug, but begins by asking himself why the bodily machinery in this particular patient is wearing out in this particular manner, and then proceeds to take the case in the manner peculiar to homoeopathy, i.e. a careful and close questioning about the patient's symptoms, because through those symptoms the body emphatically proclaims, in a way which is only understandable to the homoeopath, its urgent and insistent needs. There is a general wearing out of the bodily machinery which the homoeopath can put right with patient skill, a skill unfortunately not possessed by his orthodox colleague, because it is not included in his curriculum. The skilled homoeopath will patiently build up in his record a picture of his patient's constitutional state, which is something quite different from the particular ailment the patient is suffering from, and this will enable him to find the *constitutional remedy* for that patient, which when found, will not only repair, renew and rejuvenate the bodily machinery in a most remarkable way, but will at the same time cure the long-standing complaint for which he has sought advice.

Herein with this wonderful power to rejuvenate is just one of the great advantages which Homoeopathy has over orthodox treatments.

CHAPTER 4

The Individuality of Man and of Medicines

'There is therefore, no other possible way in which the peculiar effects of medicines on the health of individuals can be accurately ascertained — there is no surer, no more natural way of accomplishing this object, than to administer the several medicines experimentally, in moderate doses, to healthy persons, in order to ascertain what changes, symptoms and signs of their influence each individually produces on the health of the body and of the mind.'

ORGANON, Para. 108.

This is the plan introduced by Hahnemann, by which we are to positively ascertain the "peculiar effects of medicines" and also what individual sickness each will cure. Is it not remarkable that the Creative Power has made no two men alike? — and equally worthy of our notice is the fact that the Creator of therapeutic agents has made no two natural medicines alike. Each man and each medicine has an individuality; and by this we distinguish one man from another and one medicine from another.

Individuality of the Patient

The individuality of the healthy man is marked by individual characteristics, manners, tone of voice, colour of the face, etc., but what we mean by the *patient's* individuality is this: the peculiar, unusual, characteristic symptoms which he has, which mark his individual sickness, in contradistinction to those which only indicate the diagnostic name of his malady.

The symptoms by which a diagnosis is made are not the sole symptoms upon which we base the homoeopathic prescription.

To know the nature of arthritis, asthma, of melancholia or migraine, of itself, gives no clue to their remedial treatment. The special stimulus which must be brought to bear on the economy in order to overcome its derangement and thus lead the patient's body back to healthy action, must be discovered by quite another method. Its discovery must be by a distinct process, and its administration must be guided by science and art.

The individualizing symptoms in any given sickness, must be matched by the individualizing symptoms of the medicine, if to prove curative, and here lies the secret of successful prescribing. Choosing the medicine which is homoeopathic to the individual sickness. A medicine can be specific only for the individual case; and he who can grasp with accuracy the individual image of sickness possesses a sure guide.

Referring to this subject, Hahnemann said, '*Without the most minute individualization, Homoeopathy is not conceivable.*'

The founder of Homoeopathy, throughout his work, took every opportunity to urge the insufficiency of pathological prescribing. A prescription based upon a pathological consideration only, must forever prove futile, because if such were possible, it must depend upon the correctness of the pathological hypothesis — a matter in which no man can be certain. On the other hand, the trained homoeopath can discern symptoms and signs of individual sickness without speculation; and the only sure indication for every case is found in the totality of these signs and symptoms which each case presents.

When Hahnemann said '*The most minute individualization*' he did not shade the picture too delicately.

Let the similar remedy be always found for the existing symptoms and the conditions of each individual case.

Let those symptoms be the principal ones — the peculiar, striking and unusual ones.

Let the remedy be given which has as its own characteristics the characteristics of the patient.

Let it be given in the highly dynamized and purest form.

It is well enough that the selected remedy has the particular form of structural disease we are faced with, but it is far more important that it has all the constitutional and individualizing symptoms and conditions of the patient.

CHAPTER 5

If Everyone Had Their Constitutional Remedy

It is a common saying that there is no absolute on this earth and therefore no norm of complete health. Those who are familiar with Hahnemann's theory of the chronic miasms have some basis for understanding why this is so. A new born baby carries the cumulative load of ill health of all its ancestors, and the adult adds to this the weight of pernicious drugs, bad hygiene and habits and the sequels of whatever diseases he has had, including the physical and emotional resultants of mental stress. Let anyone who is financially or mathematically minded, figure out the sum total of these liabilities, which have been compounding over many years, and they will be appalled at the apparently insoluble bankruptcy as to health, of every human being.

Sensible living, sociological and emotional adjustments, abidance by the laws of spiritual life, and the correct cure of acute diseases by homoeopathic remedies, will do something toward alleviating this condition, but these measures will be palliative and preventive only, if they are not connected with chronic constitutional medication in accordance with the law of similars.

What do we mean by the *Homoeopathic chronic constitutional remedy*? We mean that substance (medicine) which is similar to the totality of symptoms, mental, emotional and physical, of our patient. We must take into consideration not only the present status, but also all shocks, illnesses, crises and tendencies in the life of our patient and in so far as we can ascertain it, in the parents and ancestors. We must review the whole career of our patient from the time of conception.

With all this complicated history, can we reasonably expect to find one remedy which will be similar to such a galaxy of symptoms? In many patients, yes. We will clearly see how the appalling headaches better by binding up the head, from which our patient suffers today, are the logical outcome of his condition in childhood, with his terror of thunderstorms, his foetid foot sweat, his dislike of milk, his lack of stamina. In such a case, one dose of *Silica* in moderate potency (200 or IM) may commence to turn our patient into order *from within outwards, from above downwards, and in the reverse order of the symptoms*, the habitual headaches giving place to the return of perspiration which in turn disappears, leaving our patient better balanced, more resistant and *less likely to have future illness of any sort.*

In the majority of cases, however, it is not so simple. One must, as it were, work back through layer after layer of engrafted and inherited disease by means of a series, not only of potencies of the same remedy but of several remedies, often related, one after the other.

This is the age of prevention, of organised effort to get the children early and protect them. Let us make a special effort to prescribe fundamentally for patients of *every age.*

To those of you who use mainly acute remedies, to those of you who shape your case-taking to fit the few polycrests you are most familiar with, I say — look into this matter of chronic treatment, study your Hahnemann's *Chronic Diseases,* Von Grauvogl's *Text Book of Homoeopathy, Kent's Lectures on Homoeopathic Philosophy,* and realise the tremendous value of giving every child and most adults their *chronic constitutional remedy,* the unit dose, repeated at intervals when the self feels worse (patient less well) and symptom progress in accordance with Hering's three rules has ceased.

The scales are before your eyes, in one, balance the cumulative tendencies to disease including excessive temperaments, in the other balance the power of the *constitutional remedy.*

Sometimes steadily, sometimes swiftly, the balance will fall on the side of the remedy and your patient will be animated by the flood tide of returning health.

CHAPTER 6

Successful Homoeopathic Prescribing

What constitutes a successful homoeopathic prescription is not thoroughly comprehended, by many who use the words.

Firstly: Only the prescriptions which are carefully selected for an individual patient as one organism, disturbed in harmony — one being, in which every disturbance is but a manifestation of the internal disorder, and then only when the selection is based on the similarity between the patient's disorder and that which the homoeopathic remedy is capable of curing. Equally opposed to the fundamental doctrines of scientific prescribing are selection of a remedy according to the symptoms manifested by one or more parts of the body without reference to their relation to the entire sick patient, and selection of a remedy because of the name of the disorder present, regardless of the peculiar individual characteristics present. Homoeopathy insists first, last, and always, that *the health of the patient*, as an individual and a unit, *is the paramount consideration* — the parts involved and the name of the disorder being secondary.

Secondly: Only the prescriptions which help to restore the patient to more harmonious mental and physical activity, with increase of power and strength from one year to the next can be admitted to be successful. We look into the work wrought for a reply when the question of success arises, not into the market or the patronage. This was Emerson's measure of happiness. This, indeed is the one great reason that Homoeopathy has held sway through the years and is now widely disseminated throughout the world. This is the only reason it is worth the attention of its adherents or those, who in their lack of knowledge criticise — because it affords this success. The pleasant doses, easy to take, the economy, arising from paying less for the medicine: the milder manner of recovery from acute disorders; all these would not suffice as reasons for its adoption or its rejection, were it not for the change in strength, power and freedom from repeated or continued suffering which it affords. Administration of medicines according to the doctrines of Homoeopathy is the only form of medical treatment, in all history, that has held out hope or given the experience of banishment of ills to which the patient has been subject, together with general increase of healthful activity. The concern of the homoeopath delving into the healing art, is how such successful prescribing may be attained. How can we learn to duplicate the wonderful results of the master-prescribers — results that win the gratitude of those who are personally benefited and the admiration of all lovers of success?

While the attainment is not the work of a day or a year, every prescriber can become a master-prescriber just in proportion to his will — his desire for success and will to follow in the paths which the masters have trod. By steadfastly following the methods Hahnemann used in the doctrines he presents in THE ORGANON, CHRONIC DISEASES, and MATERIA MEDICA PURA; by continuously and persistently refraining from substituting any methods in practice antagonistic to those doctrines, each earnest student will develop the faculty, attain the art, and win the reward.

Careful search for the personal remedy to each patient who attends for treatment serves to increase familiarity with the remedies with their distinguishing differences. The mind is thus trained to perceive the image of a remedy in even the complex forms of disorder. Continuous study of the remedies and meditation on the action observed to follow their accurate application, according to the Law, develops the master-mind able to make curative prescriptions that were impossible in the earlier years of his work.

The master-prescriber perceives here an image of *Nat. Sulph*; there, a *Ferrum phos*; in another, *Tuberculinum, Argentum nit.*, or *Kali-ars*. The less proficient one demands to know the symptoms in the record which reveal the remedy. Sometimes the strong lines may be traced in the peculiar general and particular symptoms, but sometimes the image is perceived without defining separate lines, and the answer is given: 'It is the entire patient — the entire record; — study the remedy and see it for yourself.'

Such perception cannot be transmitted nor revealed to another so that he can use it. It must be inherently developed in the student by his own application. When the successful prescriber is asked 'How do you do it?' he can reply 'By following the doctrines. This is the way. Walk in it.'

CHAPTER 7

Selection of the Indicated Remedy by Use of the Repertory

This subject is a vast one and difficult to understand correctly. Its channels of progression are various, and its number of failures corresponds in direct ratio to a faulty understanding of Materia Medica and lack of comprehension of the laws stated in THE ORGANON and in THE CHRONIC DISEASES. One may think it easy to select the indicated remedy by use of the Repertory, but it requires much exacting study.

It is utterly impossible to use the Repertory intelligently without becoming thoroughly grounded in the laws and fundamental principles of Homoeopathy.

The first, and probably the most difficult problem, is to obtain the true characteristic symptoms of the case. Every true homoeopath will admit that the recording of symptoms is difficult. Some patients are averse to giving a full symptomatic picture, while others will say so much and reveal so little that it is almost impossible to determine which of the symptoms recited actually depict the case.

In the former instance, delay formal preparation or *arrangement of the symptoms* until a sufficient number of symptoms is obtained. If these are not ascertainable from the patients direct recital, observe his demeanour, attitude and appearance when he visits your rooms, and in the meantime obtain as much information as may be available from next of kin. In reciting his case, nearly every patient will dwell upon some certain phase of his ailment. If this is characteristic of the patient and not of some classified disease, it will be of value to include it in the ultimate enumeration.

As to the patient who says so much and reveals so little, his immediate family can often furnish a much clearer image of his disorder than he does. Your own observation and a withholding of judgement until a sufficient number of characteristic symptoms is registered will mark the only safe course of procedure.

In investigating a case, the homoeopath should avoid the direct questioning which evokes the answer 'Yes' or 'No', but should tactfully lead the patient to tell his story in his own language. Hahnemann gives explicit directions upon this subject in his Explanatory Remarks appended to THE ORGANON.

Assuming that the record of the case is properly taken, the symptoms obtained must then be arranged in the order of their importance. Symptoms that are common to the disease present but are not characteristic of any individual remedy or group of remedies are of little or no value to be carried through the Repertory study. *The strongest characteristic symptoms of the patient* should appear first upon the list, followed by the next strongest, and so on down, the particular symptoms, i.e. those relating to a part and not predicated by the whole, being last considered, as being of the least value. Common symptoms add nothing for remedy selection.

After the case has been worked out, there is yet to be selected from the remedies thereto related — *the most similar remedy.* One must keep in mind that it is not always the remedy that runs numerically the highest in the grading that should be selected, but *the one which furnishes the image most similar to the picture of the entire case.*

The homoeopath should know his remedies as the botanist the plant forms, otherwise he will be unable to determine the indicated remedy. For example: one unfamiliar with the characteristics of *Cyclamen* is not able to choose between it and *Pulsatilla,* because of their many similarities. To use the Repertory intelligently and with profit, the homoeopath should study his Materia Medica (the provings of his many medicines), for its thorough acquaintance. Then the Repertory will be of inestimable value in selecting the medicines that are to be considered for the need of the individual case. When not previously familiar with the remedies to which the Repertory directs attention, the prescribing must refer to the proving records of the individual remedies.

Many cases cannot be worked out with the Repertory and the remedy must be selected by the homoeopath's knowledge, his most precious possession, an intimate acquaintance with many different remedies.

One must remember that the Repertory is only one of many requisites for efficient work of the true homoeopath. The use of the Repertory should be undertaken only after gaining an intimate knowledge of the characteristics of the various remedies, and should then be developed only as an aid in eliminating from consideration the dissimilar medicines, narrowing down the list to the few similar ones from which to select the one indicated, *the most similar remedy.*

CHAPTER 8

Repertory Study

To use the Repertory successfully, depends on ability to grade and evaluate symptoms correctly, and this has to be taught.

To show which symptoms are of vital importance to the correct prescription; which are of less importance and which may be safely used as *eliminative* symptoms. This subject has been covered so thoroughly and so frequently through the years that it would appear presumptuous of me to present it again. But it is surprising how many are not perfectly familiar with the correct procedure for repertory study.

The strength of Homoeopathy has always depended on the thorough training of her followers in knowledge of the philosophy, together with an intelligent use of the repertory. Successful study and use of the repertory is impossible apart from a study and knowledge of philosophy of Homoeopathy. The fact has been observed that those who are disappointed in repertory work are those who have neglected to study the principles set forth in *The Organon*.

Naturally, almost the first inquiry of the beginner in taking up this study is: What repertory is best adapted to meet the requirements of the homoeopathic prescriber? Whilst I am familiar with Boenninghausen's and would not be without it, I do not hesitate to declare Kent's Repertory to be superior to all others.

First: Its construction conforms to the Hahnemannian idea of Patient, in the arrangement of symptoms; from general to particular groups.

Second: It follows the Hahnemannian schema, also, of working from Mind to Generalities, thence to Particulars or parts.

Third: It is self-indexed, and to anyone who will take time to familiarise himself with its general form or plan of construction, it is simplicity itself for finding symptoms sought. There is enormous information encompassed within its covers, in a form easily obtained.

Case Recording

We must never allow our knowledge of repertory work to lead us to neglect the art of accurate, reliable case-taking, with the greatest attention to detail. Many fall here, at the starting point and are surprised and disappointed when the prescription fails, even though careful repertory study was employed.

One difficulty in this must be recognised. It is true that in these days of drugging when more and more drugs are given and less and less is understood about the patient, when seriously damaging side effects engraft themselves on the very constitution of the patient and finally that patient in his misery decides to try Homoeopathy, we meet many obscure cases presenting only a few common symptoms and repertory study can guide us only to a group of remedies in which the *similimum* must be found after further questioning of the patient and closer study of individual remedies in the materia medica.

Sometimes in these obscure cases we may find the needed remedy by *going back into past history*, at times even back to childhood, proceeding from, and through adult life, noting the signs and symptoms that appeared long before ultimates or pathology came to clog the free expression of deranged health, and before pernicious drugs were given which mask and stifle the case by implanting their own side effects on the already sick patient.

Having taken the case in accordance with the directions of Hahnemann as clearly laid down in *The Organon*, we are then prepared to analyse it for repertory study, and just here a knowledge of philosophy is of value, to indicate *the relative value of symptoms*, for selecting the proper rubrics with which to start the study.

Symptoms to be Used

We are taught that the mind symptoms *when well marked and constituting a deviation from the normal of the patient* are of the highest value in *helping* to select the indicated remedy. The mind symptoms, from the *degrees of value* may be divided into three groups.

A. The first group comprises those of the will, manifesting perversions of the loves (affections), together with the various fears.

These are the most interior, and are often concealed from the physician, as also from the world in general, but when obtained, are of the highest possible value in selection of the proper medicine.

Next in point of value are perversions of the understanding or intellect, manifesting illusions, hallucinations, delirium etc.

The third group embraces perversions of the memory which are of lowest value among the mental symptoms.

All of the foregoing symptoms are to be found in the repertory in the section of MIND.

B. Next in order are the physical generals which manifest the physical loves and the sensations of the body as a whole.

The highest in rank among these are perversions in the *sexual sphere*. Taking the normal as our guide any *excess, decrease* or *perversion* constitutes a symptom.

We need to consider the normal and its limits, in relation to the patient, that we may recognise what is abnormal or disease. The sexual symptoms are found in the repertory under GENITALIA.

Next are the symptoms pertaining to the appetite, food desires and aversions, found under STOMACH, because appetites are manifested through the stomach.

C. Then following the responses to things affecting the entire physical body; weather and climatic influences, and extremes of temperature, found in GENERALITIES. Foods that aggravate are also listed in this section because the entire patient is affected by them.

D. Any symptoms which the personal pronoun 'I' is used to describe, are general symptoms.

Haemorrhages and discharges from the body are, in their nature, general, because the organism as a whole is concerned in their elaboration.

E. After considering the generals in the order above named, we take the symptoms pertaining to the various parts of the body; head, extremities, chest etc., found in the special Part sections of the repertory. These are known as particulars and are of lower value than the physical generals.

Extending through all these symptoms from the innermost to the outermost, from mind to skin, from general to particulars, we must distinguish two grand divisions:

a. *The strange, rare, peculiar and therefore uncommon.*

b. Those that are common.
   Symptoms that are: Common to provings of many remedies
                      Commonly found in certain diseases
                      (diagnostic)
                      Common to nearly all illnesses
   are of very low value. Be they general or particular, mental or physical, they must be considered last in every case of sickness when the correct prescription is desired.

It is best to start the repertory study of a case with a general group of remedies and proceed to the more particular. For example; a symptom of pain referred to the fingers may not be found at all under the heading Fingers, but the same pain or sensation will probably be found under Hand. The method of procedure to be followed throughout the entire work is to take the broad general group first, then work through to the more particular.

As general groups belonging to the class of Common Symptoms are of less value, of course, if one of these be selected, considerably more work is necessary to attain the desired end: viz., the remedies or remedy extending all through the case.

I give you the following typical case which is sufficiently full of repertory study to illustrate working to a single remedy.

Mrs. C. aged 46 years. Headaches constant, worse lying; occipital pain, sense of pressure. Dizziness and dimness of vision. Difficult breathing when ascending stairs, and when leaning back. Sighs much recently. Sleep good at night, but tired in the morning; wants to sleep all the time; worse after eating. Hungry but easily satisfied. No thirst. Flatus considerable. Very restless. Sadness from music. Memory poor. Speech stuttering recently. Concentration difficult. Imagines she sees things running across the floor, mice etc. Thinks of nothing but death. Homesick, whenever way visiting. Irritable and cross. Sensitive to noise. Desires company. Better in open air, must have it. Very sensitive to tight collars and tight clothing anywhere. Urination frequent; copious, worse when on her feet. Menstrual period irregular; delayed, at times two or three months; flow copious 3 or 4 days; discharge very dark, strong odour, excoriating during latter part of period.

We will start with delusions (imaginations, hallucinations, illusions) and because of the *strength* of this symptom will take only those remedies in black type and italics. Remember that the *degree* or *intensity* of a symptom must also be taken into consideration and here can be used as an *eliminative symptom*.

Now before we go any further! The theory of the eliminative symptom is this: We cannot consider all the remedies in the materia medica and for practical purposes we try to limit our study, in relation to any particular case, to perhaps not more than 30 or 40 medicines, from the many hundreds we possess. The eliminative symptom does this for us, and gives us immediately a list of medicines to start with.

But remember this: An eliminative symptom must have two attributes —

(1) It must be the proper size, that is, it must not have too many remedies in it.
(2) It must be a symptom which expresses the patient, a symptom which is a particular feature of that person's reaction to the disease in question.

Practically I find that a good mental, a general modality, or a rare symptom is all sufficient. Invariably the student makes one or the other of the following mistakes. He either selects a symptom which has a hundred or more remedies in it, or he picks out a fine individual symptom which has so few remedies in its small rubric that the real similimum will be eliminated from the start.

Mentals

Delusions etc. *Acon., Aeth., Ambr., ARG-N., Ars., Aur., Aur-mur., Bapt., BELL., Calc., Camph., CANN-I., Cann-s., COCC., Coff., Glon., HYOS., IGN., Kali-br., LACH., Lyc., Merc., Nit-ac., Op., PETR., PHOS.AC., Phos., Plat., Psor., Puls., Rhus-t., SABAD., Sec., Sil., Staph., STRAM., SULPH., Valer., Zinc.*

Desires Company: Aeth., ARG-N., ARS., Aur.m., Bell., *Calc., Camph.,* HYOS., *Ign.,* Kali-br., LYC., Merc., PHOS., *Puls.*

Sensitive to noise: *Arg-n., Ars.,* BELL., *Calc.,* Camph., Hyos., *Ign., Lyc.,* Merc., Phos., Puls.

Sadness from music — (Sensitive to music) *Lyc.,* Merc., *Phos.*

Physical Generals

Open air ameliorates — ARS., *Camph., Hyos., Lyc., Phos.,* PULS.

Restless — ARS., CAMPH., HYOS., LYC., Phos., PULS.

Menstrual flow irregular — Hyos., Lyc., Phos., Puls.

Menstrual flow dark — *Ars.,* Lyc., PULS.

Tight clothing aggravates — LYC., *Puls.*   LYC 10m cured.

Analysis

The mechanical side of this working out shows LYC and PULS competing for pride of place, but the artistic side, as it has been called, that is when these two remedies are taken to the Materia Medica for further comparison with the balance of the case, quickly reveals LYCOPODIUM to be the SIMILIMUM.

To continue, the most important general here, is the derangement of the rational sphere, where the imagination holds temporary sway, but not to the extent of insanity, for the patient is yet aware that it is only an illusion that affects her. *Imagine that she sees mice and insects running across the floor etc.*

We begin with Imagination/Delusions (in general) because it is the broadest rubric on the subject and it cannot be omitted from the remedy; the required remedy *must* be in this group.

If we start with *delusions of animals or of mice or of insects* we might omit the remedy needed by the patient, since many special symptoms have not yet been observed and recorded in detail, even in the thoroughly proved remedies.

Think of Synonyms; select the rubric *containing the largest list of remedies or broadest in scope*. Get a book of synonyms if necessary and select good synonyms. If you use synonyms be sure that they are synonyms and cannot be perverted and remember that you are always working with similars.

Professor Kent in Homoeopathic Philosophy Lecture XXIII clearly states '*in general terms you can substitute terms of expression so long as you do not change the idea*'.

Another thought arises that is available when starting study of a case; we can save much work by bearing in mind that the remedy which is to be prescribed must correspond to the sickness, not only in symptomatology, but also in nature. For a chronic case, it is folly to consider remedies that relate to acute conditions, and are superficial and of short duration in action, although they extend through the symptoms of the case. They may palliate for a while, but they cannot cure, and *will only spoil the case by changing the image*.

From the record just cited, one might conclude that only a case completely recorded, or one containing striking and uncommon symptoms is suitable for repertory-study. In fact the reverse of this is true. Cases, especially of long standing disorders, and I see many of them, cases that have had much drugging, many treatments, and now present but few common symptoms, often will yield an astonishing result, through careful repertory study when other methods have failed to bring satisfaction. A brief case will illustrate.

Mrs Y. aged 42 years. Constipation for the past year; must take drugs, and then has diarrhoea. Has lost 12 or 14 lbs in the past month. Headache frequently; with nausea and vomiting, worse by rest; head better after vomiting. Vertigo with head pain. Stomach: Aversion to milk and eggs; to all foods; vomits everything eaten and drunk almost immediately after taking into stomach, even water. Mind: Irritable; worse noise, very sensitive to noise; loathing of everything in life; apathetic, much unhappiness and trouble. Menstruation — every two weeks with pain; discharge copious, dark even to black.

The remedy was worked out as follows —

27

Sensitive to noise — ACON., *Arg.n.*, *Arn.*, *Ars.*, *Ars.i.*, ASAR., *Aur.*, *Bar.c.*, BELL., BOR., *Bry.*, *Calc.*, *Carb.s.*, *Carb.v.*, *Caust.*, *Cham.*, CHIN., China.A., *Cocc.*, COFF., CON., *Ferr.*, *Ferr.ar.*, *Ferr.p.*, *Fl.ac.*, *Hell.*, *Ign.*, *Ip.*, KALI.C., *Kali-p.*, *Lac.c.*, *Lach.*, *Lyc.*, *Lyss.*, *Mag.m.*, *Med.*, *Merc.*, *Nat.c.*, *Nat.m.*, *Nat.s.*, NIT.AC., NUX.V., OP., *Phos.*, *Plat.*, *Puls.*, SEP., SIL., *Spig.*, THER., ZINC.

Irritability is so common we refer immediately to stomach symptoms.

Aversion to milk — *Arn.*, Bell., *Bry.*, *Calc.*, *Carb.v.*, Ferr.p., *Ign.*, NAT.C., Nux.v., *Phos.*, *Puls.*, *Sep.*, *Sil.*

Vomiting after drinking — *Arn.*, Bell., BRY., Calc., Ferr.p., *Nux.v.*, PHOS., Puls., *Sil.*

Menses frequent — Arn., BELL., BRY., CALC., NUX-V., PHOS., Puls., *Sil.*

Menses dark — Arn., *Bell.*, *Bry.*, *Calc.*, Ferr.p., NUX-V., PULS.

Menses copious — *Arn.*, BELL., *Bry.*, CALC., Ferr-p., NUX-V., *Puls.*

Diarrhoea after cathartics — NUX-V.

Here we have worked readily to NUX-V., and the results were amazing in a very short time. The improvement has been constant including increase in weight and strength.

The mental symptoms of indolence and irritability rapidly disappeared.

The remedy was prescribed but twice, six weeks apart, in the 10m potency.

Grades of Remedies

For beginners I direct attention to the three types used for names of remedies throughout the repertory.

1st. The Capital type records the remedies that brought out the symptoms in many provers and have been verified by repeatedly curing.

2nd. The *italics* are a grade lower. These have been noted in fewer provers, yet having been verified by cures, are reliable.

3rd. The remedies in common type have been observed to cause the symptoms in only a few provers or the symptoms were observed clinically. They are somewhat doubtful or, of lower grade in ascertained value.

Summary

A few hints in summarising this important subject.

1. Study and practice the art of *taking the case*. Even endeavour to improve this vitally important aspects of the homoeopathic art.

2. Do not hope to obtain the *fullest* use of the repertory without a study and a thorough understanding of the philosophy of Homoeopathy.

3. *Grade the relative value of symptoms* when starting the repertory study of any case, acute or chronic.

4. In cases expressed largely in common symptoms do not expect the repertory to guide you to the single remedy, work to the smallest group you can reach and then consult the materia medica for the similimum.

5. When you fail to find a symptom in the language of the patient do not despair but try some synonym. We are working continually in similars!

6. It is pointed out that great polychrests like *Sulphur, Calcarea, Lycopodium* etc., will run high in any repertory study, due to their tremendous number of symptoms so be sure it is 'degree' totality, not simply numerical and always consult the materia medica to corroborate your selection.
    To repeat. It is not so much a numerical totality, as it is a *'degree of intensity'* totality.

This is but a synopsis of the work that has been much better outlined in the Lectures on Homoeopathic Philosophy; but repetition, even in rugged from is often necessary, to impress the essentials of a subject.

CHAPTER 9

Finding the Remedy

The following appeal for assistance in Repertory-work is here answered by Edward Cotter and it is hoped that this detailed analysis will be of help to many in the difficult task of Grading and Classifying cases for Repertory Study.

Q. Dr. — writes: 'I am puzzled to know when to call a symptom usually classed as particular, a general.'

(1) Would constant coldness on top of the head (requiring covering and warmth) although a particular become general?

(2) A patient complains of: Chronic (dry, scaly) eczema of lower extremities as far as the hips, of many years duration; also: Haemorrhoids (piles) protruding during stool. These two troubles he has had for six or seven years. These both are particular; would they, in this case, form the basis for repertory study, and thus become generals?

(3) He is also much benefited by a bath (bathing ameliorates), both generally and locally and the eczema is slightly improved. As bathing is normal to all people and should ameliorate, it might be a common general symptom, but in this case would you call it *rare, strange, peculiar* and therefore include it as one of the main symptoms *which cannot be omitted*, or even a basic symptom for repertory-study?

(4) He is also lacking in vital heat. Has a strong tendency to catch cold in winter. Has coldness at back of head and neck, knees, thighs. Must keep covered, at night even a part of head covered, to keep warm.

I write *Lack of vital heat* as a basic symptom (because *Uncovering aggravates* would not necessarily cover this feature). He complains of cold when he uncovers, but this would also aggravate, so I use both these generals for 'rare' symptoms which cannot be omitted. If one of these symptoms is superfluous, which would you omit?

He has flushes of heat.

Is easily embarrassed in company, or timid.

Bowels move before breakfast, motions soft.

My arrangement is as follows:—

> (1) Timidity. (2) Lack of vital heat. (3) Disposition to
> cold. (4) Uncovering aggravates. (5) Flushes of heat. (6)
> Chronic, dry, scaly, slightly itching eczema. (7) Haemorr-
> hoids protruding during stool. (8) Amelioration from
> bathing. (9) Coldness; back of neck, knees, thighs. (10)
> Covering part of head, at night.

(5) I would take symptoms 1, 2 and 8 as basic symptoms, for
working out the others. If eczema and haemorrhoids
come in as generals, they may have to be included for
repertory study.

By actual count I found *Silica* to be the remedy. I
desire, in this case, to know the proper grouping for
repertory study.

A. (1) (*Ans.*) Not when related to a single part. But a sensation
of either heat or coldness related to many parts of the
body is then a general feature of the case and must be
used as a general symptom. However, it is but a common
one because such symptoms are common to many drug-
provings and are generally in many complaints.

(2) (*Ans.*) They cannot become generals because they are
related only to special parts: viz. the skin of the lower
extremities, and the mucous membrane and inferior
haemorrhoidal veins of the rectum.

If you had no generals in the case and no other particulars of great value, they might form the basis for repertory study, but you would work to quite a large group of
remedies, and would only come to the single remedy by
further study of the materia medica. Probably closer
observation and questioning of your patient would be
necessary before an intelligent prescription could be
made.

(3) (*Ans.*) The patient as a whole ameliorated by bathing is a
general symptom, but of low grade value because it is
common. The skin condition relieved by bathing

although a particular, is somewhat uncommon because most chronic skin conditions are aggravated by bathing, though this is far from universal.

However, any skin symptom is of minor importance in making a homoeopathic prescription, because the skin corresponds to the patient's externals and therefore belongs to the low grade physical generals. It might be as well to inquire about hot and cold bathing here.

(4) (*Ans.*) In these questions you have succeeded beautifully in bringing out the fact that the patient is a decidedly chilly one, and is aggravated from cold in general.

(5) (*Ans.*) The symptoms you mention, viz: 1, 2 and 8 are all right to begin the case or as a basis but then to be followed by 5 and 3.

These symptoms with the rather uncommon particular symptoms of coldness referred to the head are sufficient to work to Psorinum. Please observe that Silica is aggravated by bathing, getting wet, etc., and consequently is not a complete similar.

I append my working out of this case, for your guidance.

Timidity (compare bashfulness and fear in general):
Am-m., Ars., Aur., BAR-C., *Bor.,* CALC., CALC-S., *Carb-s., Caust., Chin., Coca., Con.,* GELS., *Graph., Ign., Kali-ar.,* KALI-C., *Kali-s.,* LYC., *Merc., Nat-a.,* NAT-C., *Nat-m., Nux-v.,* PETR., PHOS., PLB., *Puls., Rhus-t.,* SEP., *Sil., Stram.,* SULPH.

Lacks vital heat:
Alu., ARS., *Am-m.,* BAR-C., CALC., *Carb-s.,* CAUST., *Chin., Con.,* GRAPH., KALI-ARS., KALI-C., *Lyc., Merc., Nat-a.,* NUX-V., PSOR., *Petr.,* PHOS., *Plb.,* RHUS-T., *Sep.,* SIL., *Sulph.*

Bathing ameliorates:
Alum., Am-m., Caust. Psor.

Heat flushes:
Alum., Caust., Psor.

Tendency to take cold:
ALUM., *Caust.,* PSOR.

Head sensitive to cold:
   Psor.

Uncovered aggravated:
   Psor.

You will notice that *timidity* does not come through the working out and this is where an intimate knowledge of Materia Medica is indispensable. Those who are familiar with the *anxiety* and *fear* found under Psorinum, will immediately see the diminutive in *timidity*, and in relation to the balance of the case.

N.B. — *This question was received some time ago and dealt with personally. The writer has since had the pleasure of learning that a perfect cure was affected by Psorinum 10m.*

CHAPTER 10

Therapeutic and General Hints

If after long treatment of a chronic case good reaction is not forth-coming take all the general and significant symptoms from the beginning to the end of the record and base a prescription on them.

Mark down Kali Mur is your repertories under 'Pain in throat relieved by cold drinks'. It is most positive. *Phos.* is another; *Kali-bi.* also, at times.

Lycopodium 30 is a wonderful acting chronic remedy.

For bronchial pneumonia, if only partial response to apparently well indicated remedies, think of *Tuberculinum.*

Try Alum., low, for constipation of infants fed on baby-food.

Septic wounds in which *Lachesis* is indicated may have the pain relieved by cold the first few days but not longer.

Strontium-carb. should be thought of more often in connection with surgical shock. Study it.

Before major operation procedure do not forget the beneficial effect of a dose of *Phosphorous* 200 the night before the opera-tion.

When *All-cep.* is the acute remedy, *Phos.* will be complemen-tary and the *chronic*, quite often.

Merc. protoiod 6x for follicular tonsilitis, look closely before you think of another.

Hydrangea arborescens in uncomplicated enlargement of the elderly prostate gland; five to ten drops, night and morning, long continued.

Complaints which rouse the patient from sleep are often calling for *Medorrhinum*, and not always for one of the ophidia.

Remember that in whooping cough *Drosera* has a puffy face as well as *Kali-carb.*

For patients whose only symptom is waking early in the morn-ing and being unable to go to sleep again, think not only of *Sulph*, but also of *Bellis-per.*

For the dizziness of cerebral stasis in old people, think again of *Bellis-per.*

In sex difficulties of women at the mid-century think of *Medor-rhinum* or *Lueticum*; or, if spasms are present and the patient wakes in the night with lascivious thoughts, consider *Lyssin.*

In any haemorrhage, where there is no peculiar symptom indicating another remedy, give *Millefolium*.

Nux-Vomica is not a long acting stomach remedy, but does act for a long time on the central nervous system.

Remember, after an operation, even the slightest, the element of shock must be included in the totality of symptoms.

Belladonna does not bear repetition. It must never be repeated in high potency, by the inexperienced.

Remedies act particularly well during pregnancy, also a few days prior and immediately after menstruation.

In chronic cases to not repeat or change your remedy too soon — wait.

CHAPTER 11

Remedies Related to Pathological Tissue Changes

Provings of remedies are not continued to the extent of producing tissue alterations — indurations, infiltrations, suppurations, caries etc. Most of the indications for the use of remedies in these conditions have been learned clinically. When a remedy has been prescribed for a patient in whom tissue changes have occurred, the prescription being based on the symptom image, resolution of the existing tissue changes has occurred, as a result of the response to the remedy. These become reliable clinical symptoms of the remedy; demonstrations of the power of the remedy over the altered tissue. These remedies are then recognised to be suited to constitutions in which these pathological changes can develop. Hence they are as important to the prescriber as though they had appeared actually in the proving. In many instances such cure of pathology has occurred as a delightful surprise to the homoeopath, who realises in this evidence the accuracy of the prescription, which not only restored the functional activities but altered the nutrition to the extent of removing the *products of disorder.*

The difficulty in prescribing for patients with such altered tissue — cataract, hepatization (in pneumonia), induration of glands, arteriosclerosis, fibroids, tumours etc. — rests in the fact that when these tissue changes occur, the symptoms on which a prescription should be based — the symptoms of the patient have disappeared. The symptoms present at the time are symptoms of the pathology. If the symptoms that preceded this condition can be learned, and considered together with the later results of disorder — the pathological tissue — it may be possible to select a remedy that is sufficiently related to both the patient and his pathology, to effect a cure of both, providing always that the reaction and vitality of the patient are sufficient to permit the resolution.

Caust., Graph., Lyc., Nit-Ac., Staph., Thuja and many other remedies relate to excrescences. Skin indurations are met by *Ant.c., Calc. Con., Lyc., Phos., Rhus-tox., Sep., Sil., Sulph.,* and other remedies. Indurated glands find suitable remedies in *Bary-mur., Brom., Calc., Calc-f.,* and remedies of similar depth, while such remedies as *Caust., Bry., Con., Kali-c.,* and *Lyc.,* are found suitable to muscle induration. *Acon., Bapt., Gels., Ipec.,* and remedies of this scope have never been known to produce any alteration by induration and infiltration, hence the wise prescriber will not select these remedies with the aforementioned conditions, when he has those, from which to select, which are pre-eminently related to the exact condition present. The final selection of a remedy, when these conditions are present, is to be determined by the character of symptoms that preceded, or what may be present and indicative of the patient, himself.

In pneumonia, in hepatization period, when the symptoms point to *Arsenicum*, the patient will die if *Arsenicum* is given, for this remedy is not deep enough to include that infiltration. *Sulph., Lycopodium, Phosphorus, Calcarea* etc., must take up the work where *Arsenicum* could not proceed. One of these remedies will clear out the lungs, in a few hours, with a disappearance of all the symptoms dependent upon the infiltration, and the patient, freed of the burden, will be restored to health promptly, instead of succumbing to the mechanical interference and consequent air-starvation.

In arterio-sclerosis, in cataract, in induration of liver or other glandular structures, the same principle holds. *Ars., Bry., Puls.* and other short and medium acting remedies are insufficient because they have no power to take hold of this condition, while *Silica, Calcarea-fluorica, Sulph.* and such deep acting remedies have been known to remove the tissue change by the deeper action, hence are more similar, and from them, one may be selected which will prove curative.

By reference to the repertory the prescriber may find remedies which have thus been established as suitable to the deep seated disorders, with gross pathological change etc., and, as an intelligent prescriber, the homoeopath should select a remedy for the patient that is also related to the condition of the ultimate disorder. This is totally different from prescribing on the pathology alone, or seeking a specific for the name of the ultimate, regardless of the patient.

CHAPTER 12

Shock and Injury Remedies

This brief treatise in popular language has been carefully prepared to bring to the laity clear and reliable indications for the employment of some homoeopathic remedies in meeting the trauma (injuries) to mind and body which may be sustained in the daily walk of life.

It must be understood that the following remedies, few in number, have been selected to cover the immediate effects of trauma and not the complicated cases of later life which can only be unravelled by the services of those skilled to do so.

Sudden emotions — shocks to the nervous system — so often are the forerunner of more serious trouble but may be averted by timely homoeopathic prescribing. After a common *fright*, caused by a sudden noise, or ill-timed practical joke, etc., give OPIUM if it can be given immediately; but if an hour or more should have elapsed ACONITE is preferable.

After a *fright* with great *terror*, or if *fear of the fright* remains, OPIUM is the best remedy.

Fright with vexation give ACONITE; if followed by *sadness* or *grief*, give IGNATIA. If children after being frightened are still full of fear, have great heat in the head and twitching around the mouth, give OPIUM.

If the *fright* is followed by twitching of the limbs, or convulsions, insensibility, loss of sight, trembling, difficult breathing, involuntary evacuations give OPIUM; and if this should have no effect within half an hour give IGNATIA or GLONOINE as one of these should help.

If children have been frightened into *fits*, and scream, tremble, with twitching in the arms and legs — if the head is hot, with much perspiration and redness of face, give OPIUM every 5 or 10 minutes; if not better in half an hour BELLADONNA should be given; but if they become very pale IGNATIA; if very cold with involuntary evacuations VERATRUM.

In case of simple *vomiting*, sickness of the stomach, or pains caused by fright, give ACONITE.

For *diarrhoea*, caused by any sudden mental emotion, such as grief, fright, bad news, the anticipation of any unusual ordeal, give GELSEMIUM; if coldness and trembling are associated with the diarrhoea, give VERATRUM.

Grief and sorrow come to us all, sooner or later, and the consequences of these emotions, if long continued, ravage the human economy in a multitude of ways. The first sudden consequences are, however, in most cases soon overcome by medicines.

For the *grief of bereavement*, IGNATIA.

For *grief*, caused by *disappointment in love*, IGNATIA.

For *disappointed love*, with *vexation* and *anger*, STAPHISAGRIA.

If much affected by *great sympathy with the sickness or other distress* of a friend or someone near and dear, PHOS.AC.

For the lasting effects of old grief, seek professional advice.

External Injuries

And now that wonderful remedy ARNICA, so misunderstood and consequently mis-used.

ARNICA is NOT the remedy for shock, as many people think, you will find no reference to it above, but is THE *remedy* in all cases of *shock* from *external violence*.

When you think of ARNICA, think of a severe fall, blow, knock, contusion, sprain, over-stretching or laceration of the body.

I remember a bad case of rheumatoid arthritis which dated from a fall two or three years previously, completely wiped out by a high potency of ARNICA; but back to the domestic application of this beautiful remedy.

With the type of injury mentioned ARNICA lotion, i.e. 10 drops of the mother tincture to half a pint of cold water, may be advantageously employed as a moist compress and bandaged in position if possible in addition to the 30c potency internally. But the lotion should not be applied to a wound where the skin is broken.

Over-lifting. If lifting or carrying heavy loads, or any sudden exertion of strength produces pain, give RHUS-TOX. When from this cause violent, piercing pains are felt in the small of the back, which become worse on every motion of the body, give BRYONIA. If headache ensues, and RHUS-TOX will not remove it, give CALC-CARB.

Mis-steps sometimes cause pain in the limbs similar to over-lifting. They will generally be relieved by BRYONIA or RHUS-TOX; or, if the stomach is much affected, give BRYONIA or PULSATILLA.

Bumps on the heads of childen. Liberal applications of cold water, or water with a few drops of ARNICA *tincture* in it, and the internal application of ARNICA. A patient of mine — a lady of sixty years of age — slipped carrying a tea tray downstairs and sustained multiple bruising including a grossly swollen ankle. An hour later when the commotion had died down, her husband remembered some *ARNICA* 30 I had given him a few weeks earlier, and gave her several doses, then sat in amazement watching the ankle — 'it went down in twenty minutes'. ARNICA will prove a good friend to you if used correctly, i.e. on the clear-cut indications as outlined above.

Method of administration. With all the above remedies, other than the tincture, the 30c potency is recommended.

With children a good method is to dissolve two or three tablets (or pills) in a quarter tumbler of water and give two teaspoons of the mixture as a dose — give the same number of doses as with adults.

With adults give one tablet (two pills) every fifteen to thirty minutes for three or four doses. Discontinue as soon as improvement is noticed, but you may repeat again later if the improvement ceases or the patient regresses.

In all cases improvement will be swift or

(a) you have selected the wrong remedy.
(b) the case is not for domestic prescribing and skilled medical attention is required.

CHAPTER 13

Therapeutic Indications of Injuries

The best aids in the treatment of injuries resulting from blows, falls, shock, concussions, punctures, bruises, lacerations, and cuts, are the homoeopathic remedies: *Arnica, Calcarea-carb., Calcarea-phos., Calendula, Hamamelis, Hypericum, Ledum, Rhus-tox., Ruta, Staphisagria, Strontium-carb., Sulph. ac.,* and *Symphytum.* I do not wish to convey the impression that these remedies always supplant the use of the needle, the knife, and other instruments of the surgeon, but I do insist that these remedies in their proper sphere will save patients from needless suffering, mutilation, and possibly from death. With a knowledge of their indications the homoeopathic surgeon is better fortified to combat the results of injuries than without them.

Arnica Montana. (Leopard's-bane)

The average homoeopath knows little of this remedy, beyond the fact that it is good for falls, blows, and bruises, and that somewhere on the patient's anatomy are found 'black and blue' patches, for which *Arnica* is very useful. He freely rubs the tincture on any injury — which is quite wrong — *Arnica* must always be used diluted when applied to the skin — and should always be prepared by a thoroughly reliable homoeopathic pharmacy.

Arnica is indicated in: Bruises;
Blows;
Falls;
Shock.

Injuries to joints when there is present a marked degree of soreness; bruised soreness. Diluted *Arnica* applied externally to sprained ankle or any other joint, with a dose of the potentised substance (nothing below the 30th potency) internally will rapidly remove all effects of the sprain.

A patient, quite recently, badly bruised in a car accident. The following day lameness and soreness were felt in the entire right side. Dreamed that night several times of being killed. Pains and dreams were completely routed by a dose of *Arnica* 10M. I have seen lumps on children's heads, due to a fall, disappear very quickly after the exhibition of *Arnica* externally and internally.

The cognate of *Arnica* for ecchymosed spots ('black and blue') is *Sulph-ac.* In old people you will find that a slight blow causes a 'black and blue' patch to appear at the seat of the injury. A dose of potentised *Sulph-ac.*, will correct this condition. This remedy is very useful in bruises, boils, bedsores, injuries from falls and knocks.

In sprains of muscles, tendons and ligaments, *Arnica* must be followed by *Rhus-tox.*, particularly when the injured part is relieved by the external application of heat in any form. The usual modality of the remedy is present in such a case, i.e. the aggravation from beginning to move.

A badly treated, or neglected sprain which remains sore and weak will require *Calcarea-carb* for its eventual cure.

Calendula (Marigold)

The marigold lends itself admirably to the treatment of:
>   Lacerated wounds
>   Dental lacerations
>   Lacerations of the perinaeum
>   Any torn, jagged wound.

It very quickly heals the lacerated gums after extraction of teeth. Several of my dental surgeon friends have had abundant opportunity to verify the extraordinary healing properties of *Calendula*.

In any laceration wash the wound with a solution of one part of *Calendula* mother tincture to ten of water — this in conjunction with any surgical assistance which may be necessary.

Calcarea Phos

This preparation of *Calcarea*, when the symptoms agree, will help quickly to unite fractured ends of bones. Frequently fractures will not unite. *Calc. phos.* is one of our remedies to promote the formation of callous.

Symphytum (Comfrey)

Symphytum is another remedy to facilitate union of fractured bones by favouring the formation of callous, particularly when delay of union has nervous origin. The attending pain at seat of injury is a peculiar pricking, stitching pain.

Symphytum is used for:
>   Blow upon the eye by a tennis ball;
>   A jab into the mother's eye by an infant
>   A knock or contusion of eyes from an obtuse body inflicting a bruise.
>   Further, it will relieve the irritability of stumps after amputation.
>   Banish the periosteal pains remaining after wounds have healed.

Ruta Graveolens

Ruta is indicated for injuries of the periosteum from a fall or from any accident which causes the parts to feel very sore and bruised.
Pain as if bruised in the outer parts and in the bones.
Wounds where the bones are injured. Bruised bones.

Staphisagria (Delphinium)

What *Calendula* is for the lacerated wound, *Staphisagria* is for the clean-cut wound, by knife, razor, etc. Any incised wound calls for *Staphisagria* and is particularly suited to persons who are very sensitive to least impressions, either physical or mental. The pains are smarting and stinging in character.

Hamamelis-Virg.

Hamamelis is called for when there are sore, bruised pains in affected parts, due to incised, lacerated, contused wounds with much bleeding. The remedy checks the bleeding, removes the pains and promotes rapid healing. One of our valuable haemorrhage remedies. Often required for profusely bleeding haemorrhoids; with burning soreness in rectum. Sensation as if back would break.

Strontium carb.

Strontium-carb after a major surgical operation, with intense prostration, coldness, much oozing of blood follows, and the patient desires heat and is aggravated by the least draught of cold air. *Stront. carb.* brings wonderful comfort to this patient.

Phosphorus

Mention has been made elsewhere of the ability of *Phosphorus* to stop profuse bleeding from small wounds.
Think of this remedy for prolonged bleeding after extraction of teeth, especially in those who require cold food and drink.

Hypericum Perforatum (St. John's Wort)

Hypericum is useful for bruised and strained muscles and tendons but above all, for:
Injuries to sentient nerves.
Inflammation of nerves injured by stepping on nails, tacks, pins, splinters, even from the bite of an animal. When the pain travels

upward from the seat of the injury, and threatens tetanus (lock-jaw); where the finger ends or the toes have been bruised and lacerated or a nail torn off, or a splinter run under the nail, and the pain travels upward from the seat of the injury along the nerve toward the body, give the patient a dose of *Hypericum*, and there need be no fear of tetanus to worry you and the patient. Tetanus from wounds will not appear if the victim is given *Hypericum*.

Hypericum wounds are very *painful*: burning, stinging, shooting, throbbing pains. Open, lacerated, very painful wounds, which will not heal, often need *Hypericum*.

Neuritis from a punctured wound will be cured by the administration of *Hypericum*.

Injuries to the spine, as a fall on the coccyx, and a concussion of the spine, where the whole spine is very sensitive to touch, will respond to the potentised St. John's Wort.

Intense after pains from difficult, instrumental child-delivery, located in sacrum and hips, and are attended by severe headache. This calls for *Hypericum*, which has exhibited wonderful healing power in such a case.

Ledum Palustre (Wild Rosemary)

Ledum is another remedy for puncture wounds. Wounds made by nails, pointed instruments, strings of insects, particularly for mosquito bites. Wounds from stepping on tacks, puncturing with needles, running splinters into the hand or under the nail appear much like *Hypericum*; but when the *injured part feels cold, is puffed, pale, mottled,* give Ledum.

CHAPTER 14

Clinical Cases

The following case reports are taken directly from the records of a busy practice, they have been much abbreviated for publication, but all items of interest have been retained, and whilst these clinical cases are mainly for the profession, it is hoped they will be of interest to other readers.

Helen — age 12 years was brought to me in November 1958 with a history of nocturnal enuresis since the age of 5 years. This child had been under the care, at different times, of two well known homoeopaths in France and I learned from the mother that although the childs general health had improved wonderfully under treatment, the problem of involuntary urination remained constant.

On questioning I could elicit little of value in the nature of symptoms, which was undoubtedly due to the improvement in the patients general health; then again one is often faced with the problem of 'bed-wetting and nothing else".

However, after close interrogation I learned that the bed-wetting came on after removal of her tonsils at the age of five, these had to be removed, as, according to the mother the patient had continuous sore throats, *'first one side, then the other'*.

Lac-Caninum 10 m cured.

This case serves to show the importance of past history in homoeopathic prescribing when faced with this type of case, indeed at any time, the more especially as this patient had been in the hands of two skilled prescribers and I concluded some carefully weighed prescriptions had previously been made. I would not presume that the age at which enuresis manifested itself had escaped anyones notice but the vital clue *'first one side, then the other'* enabled this child to be cured.

John — age 7 years entered my rooms tearful and damp, it was a cold day, which no doubt lent to his discomfort. He was a well developed boy for his age, although he had suffered from an intractable catarrh since a baby. but the involuntary urination was the main complaint.

He suffered frequently from irritation of the anus but there was no history or evidence of worms. I questioned the use of aluminium cooking ware but only enamel was used. The family history was good and further questioning failed to reveal any more prescribing symptoms.   *Medhorrhinum C.M. cured.*

Patient was dry in one month and there has been no return of his tiresome complaint which was three years ago at the time of writing.

Mrs. M.R.A. age 29 years with a history of frequent miscarriages came to me in a most despondent state. It was her hearts desire to have a baby but she repeatedly aborted, once at 3 months, again at 2 months, then at 3½ months and recently at 6 weeks. Naturally she had consulted her own doctor, had been gynaecologically investigated, a dilation and curettage had been done, but all to no avail. As a last resort she had turned to homoeopathy having heard from a friend it may help her. I instructed her to take steps to prevent conception until advised to the contrary — certainly for the next 3-4 months — and then proceeded to take the case in detail.

She told me her menstrual period had always been late and during the period severe headaches were apt to occur. Prior to the period she felt gloomy and depressed. Constipation was the rule rather than the exception and the patient complained of always feeling tired. She felt nauseated in the mornings, could not take breakfast and felt depressed most of the time. *Sepia IM* was given.

May. One month later. With a smile on her face '*I feel so much better in every way*'.

June. 'My period wasn't late this time and everyone tells me I look so much better'.

July. Has gained 5 lbs in weight and says she never feels tired now, constipation completely gone and menstrual period normal.

I informed her that she may now conceive if she still so desired. The following year she gave birth to a delightful little daughter after a happy, uneventful pregnancy.

Miss G.C. a nursing sister gave the following history:

Ever since puberty she had suffered intensely during the menstrual periods. The periods were regular, but the flow was scanty, and accompanied by nausea, vomiting and diarrhoea; general coldness and dizziness and faintness. This suffering continued for two days and incapacitated her completely, leaving her very weak.

She received *Veratrum-Alb* from me during the first week following a period. She felt well during the next period and was able to continue at her work.

I had occasion to speak with this patient on the telephone regarding a patient she had sent to me, and I learnt there had been no return of the trouble and 18 months have elapsed since she was discharged.

Mr S.C.D. age 45 years had been suffering from an eczematous eruption for ten years on his hands, arms and between the thighs. He was only troubled with it during the winter months as, oddly enough, it disappeared in warm weather. Yet the itching was intensified as soon as he got warm in bed and he scratched until his skin bled, it was also aggravated by cold air and cold bathing.

Psorinum 1M immediately set this patient on the path to recovery and three winters have now passed without any return of the skin condition.

Mrs. A.H.B. age 52 years came all the way from Australia to consult me regarding her attacks of migraine, she had suffered from them for 30 years but now, during the menopause, the paroxysms of pain were intolerable, leaving the patient in an exhausted state. I at first suspected an intracranial neoplasm and was about to tell her that I would be unable to help these headaches, but, no doubt influenced by thoughts of the long journey she had made I rserved judgement and proceeded to take the case in detail. I firstly established that the aura preceeding the attacks was the same as it has always been and the unilateral character of her headaches remained unchanged, it was the intensity of the pain which had increased. Gradually the possibility of a tumour receded from my mind and a picture of the patient's symptoms took its place.

The headaches were right sided and usually started in the morning getting worse as the day wore on: light was intolerable and the only relief obtained was after vomiting, although this was not always the case and is a common symptom. The marked increase in the severity of symptoms since entering the menopause caused me to look closely into that syndrome in the hope of finding a clue but apart from generalised vaso-motor disturbances there was no other phenomena of note. But suddenly a flash of recognition crossed my mind — the particular symptoms of the migraine attacks resembled *Sanguinaria* which I had previously noted but that in itself was not sufficient authority for me to employ it, but here in the vaso-motor disturbance of the menopausal syndrome a *general feature* of *Sanguinaria* stood revealed to complete the totality of symptoms.

Sanguinaria in a series of ascending potencies steadily restored this patient and six months later when she appeared to be slipping back a little, a few doses of *Sulphur 1M* cemented her cure firmly in place.

Miss J.D., aged 27 years, recently vaccinated against smallpox prior to going abroad on holiday. The effect was dreadful. The patient presented constitutional symptoms plus a terribly swollen and inflamed arm. I regarded this case as serious and I needed a remedy to give me prompt results. In this case it was our well tried *Thuja* on the following symptoms:

Several enormous pustules

Rash on body

Diarrhoea.

High fever — (sleepless and restless for forty-eight hours)

I gave the patient one dose in the ten thousandth potency, and in two hours she quieted down, slept all night and woke in the morning free from all suffering.

Mr. A.W., aged 60 years — awakened at 8 a.m. experiencing a creeping chill in small of back. An hour later, dry burning heat, heart beats sound to him like the beat of a *drum*. Cannot lie on back or left side — without a pillow, and with *right arm stretched out behind him* to give further relief. Patient feels heart beats and they seem to him to fill the entire chest. Pulse strong and bounding, ranging from 90 to 100. Complains of much mucus flowing from back of nose. I gave one drop of a 50 per cent tincture of *Lobelia purp.* in a little water. In one minute patient felt slightly easier. I immediately gave a full drop on the tongue. In three minutes the pulse was normal; a slight perspiration broke out, and the mucus flow ceased. In fifteen minutes a natural sleep ensued, the patient waking at 2 p.m. cured.

Mr. R.W., aged 45 years, is of athletic build. Comes only for relief of belching large quantities of wind. Thinks he has heart-disease, for which he had consulted many physicians. Was addicted to alcohol, but ceased drinking six months ago. Inveterate smoker. Must always have company. Extremely restless; nervous. Choking sensation; when belching begins must leave the house and walk in the open air; impulse to jump through the window. Sight of hearse impels the imagination of skeletons, cemeteries, etc. It drives him 'crazy' to hear of dying, dead people, etc. Fear of the dark. Fear of lightning. Sleepless until 2 a.m. and restless in bed; shakes when beginning to sleep. Eructations loud and continuous after eating. Palpitation of heart — imagines it is jumping out. Stops suddenly on the street and presses hand firmly against the thorax — thinks he is about to die yet knowing this is imagination. Pulse regular. Vision cloudy, blurred. Forehead — weight appears to press down on face. Feels weak and trembling. Urination profuse and frequent during the day, or ineffectual urging.

Fleeting pains wandering quickly from place to place. Boils in the autumn — face and neck. Constipation.

Arg-Nit 200 rapidly restored this man to physical and mental health, with complete disappearance of all symptoms.

Mrs. L.D., aged 36 years, has five children. Anorexia (loss of appetite) for the past three or four years. Lives on egg-nogs. Never desires anything. Feels very chilly during the menstrual period. Has always experienced a lack of vital heat and very cold feet all her life. Skin inactive. Mentally has a dread of work, has to force herself to do things. Milk disappears two weeks after childbirth, thin while it is present and child refuses it. Menses always irregular as to time and quantity. Has been constipated since childhood.

Silica 200 was given. The very next day her appetite returned. Then slowly her constitution was turned into order. Her constipation disappeared and bowels became regular, she is now active, enjoys work, and radiates health.

Miss T.M., aged 42, qualified nurse, came to me in November, 1965, complaining of severe headaches of two years' duration. And lately they always came just prior or during the menstrual period but for the past two months they had been almost constant. Pain was concentrated on the left side of neck, left eye and down the back of the neck. Hot fomentations were found to relieve the pain in the back of the neck only. The pain was aggravated by noise, motion, stooping and when studying. Not relieved, even temporarily, by Aspirin, or other ordinary treatment. Appetite good and bowels regular. Menstrual period regular, but with scanty flow. Two years ago had a 'lot of rheumatism' which was suppressed by the use of a well advertised product. Shortly after this the headaches made their first appearance.

I gave her *Spigelia* 6 t.i.d. to discontinue them when there was some definite evidence of the headaches improving. Two weeks later she returned, delighted that the headaches were no longer with her. In June, 1966, I received a letter from her that she was taking up an appointment overseas. She has had no return of the headache, but wishes to have the name of the medicine which 'acted almost miraculously, curing my headache with two or three doses'.

Mrs S.B.J., aged 69 years, for many years a chronic sufferer of neurasthenia, migraine, rheumatic complaints, etc., on taking cold, developed what appeared to be cystitis. On account of the urging and severe burning in the neck of the bladder and the urethra, the first remedy which jumped to mind was *Cantharis*, but on continuing to carefully record the case, I found the following symptoms

Weakness in the morning.

Continuous pressure in the region of the bladder, with —

Urging to urinate when standing;

Smarting while urinating;

Sensation of heat in the lower part of the abdomen.

Much increased by motion.

In Allen's Encyclopedia we read under *Lilium Tigrinum* 'Constant burning pain across the hypogastrium from groin to groin'. This is not mentioned in Guiding Symptoms, Clarke's Dictionary nor Hering's Condensed Materia Medica, but the other symptoms of the case are all noted under this remedy.

Lilium Tigrinum 200 was given and followed by immediate improvement. A few weeks later, having become chilled, the symptoms again returned — *Lilium Tig.* 200 was given which wiped out the condition — but the most gratifying thing, which we so often find with Homoeopathy, was the tremendous benefit to her general health.

Mrs. B.M., aged 60 years, a worn-out housewife. 'So weak'. Husband says 'No company for me, always thinking about, and says she sees her dead daughter'.

On examination I found a loud systolic murmur at apex.

Ars-alb 30 was given.

Three weeks later, 'My wife is a different women since your treatment'.

Mr. R.D.A., aged 54 years, complains of frequent urination, daytime only, for past two years. Urine dark yellow, brown, watery.

Lower limbs stiff. Back easily strained. Very chilly person and particularly sensitive to cold, wet weather. Restless, must be doing something. Sleep good but deep. Periodic spells of dizziness with tendency to fall.

Rhus-tox 30. 3-times daily for two days, to report in two weeks.

Next visit — Urination less frequent. Lower limbs lighter. Report in three weeks.

Next visit — Frequent urination much better, can now go several hours without inconvenience. Urination — slow, steady; no dribbling. Wakens much refreshed. Complexion clearer, all spots and blemishes gone. Walks lightly, no heaviness in lower limbs. Feels like a new man.

Mrs. H.S.J., aged 49 years, has suffered from a liver disorder together with an aggravated form of constipation for several years and has taken many drugs which have in no way helped, and have, in fact, produced a tiresome skin rash. Realising that drugs are undermining her health she now comes to see if Homoeopathic medicines will help her.

Her symptoms are as follows:

General lassitude, malaise.

Completely fatigued from a short walk, this is even more noticeable in summer.

Hepatic region — drawing pains; pains worse lying on left side, also when waking. Dragging, pulling pain much aggravated by walking.

Transverse colon sluggish peristalsis, of which she complains much.

Stomach — a burning pain; easily deranged.

Stomach symptoms markedly aggravated by pork and greasy food.

Some palpitation.

Carduus Marianus 30 and later 200 was given. Improvement was marked and the liver responded well to treatment; she soon was able to walk miles without fatigue.

Mr. C.P., aged 46 years. Very bad attacks of migraine. Small, corpulent, haemorrhoidal, has an enormous appetite, very sleepy after eating, has renounced all sports in which he had previously excelled. He is frequently afflicted with attacks of migraine and vomiting, which confine him to bed for two or three days at a time. Pain is located in the forehead, implicating also the eyeballs. Noise, light and motion aggravate. Patient has also a most aggravated form of constipation for which he has tried various treatments, without effect. Neither his heart nor his lungs were affected. At 16 years of age he had been afflicted with an attack of renal colic. *Iris versicolor* seemed to be indicated and was prescribed in the 30th potency. After a few days he experienced an enormous evacuation and he could not recall having had such an irresistible call to stool for fifteen years. *Iris versicolor* became a precious remedy for this patient and now both constipation and migraine are things of the past.

Miss C.D., aged 21 years, presented the following symptoms: History of enteritis during the first year of infancy; later had all the eruptive diseases except scarlet fever. At twelve years tonsils were removed. First menstrual period at fourteen years with uneventful establishment. Menses now every twenty-eight days, copious for four days, last six days in all. Sadness before the menses and spells of weeping; feels better after onset of flow. Appetite fickle, is very fond of pickles, but has no other marked cravings. Bowels constipated unless some mineral oil preparation is taken. Late in falling asleep, legs jerk; talks and cries during sleep and wakes terrified; frequent nightmares. Skin cold and clammy, sensitive to cold in general; no abnormal sweats; as an infant perspired freely on the head.

Sept. *Nat. mur* 200. Three doses, four hourly intervals in one day.

Oct. 10th. A cough needed *Sanguinaria* 30.

Oct. 22nd. No mental depression before the last menstrual period, but nightmares have been a little more frequent of late.

Nat. mur. 1M. Three doses, four hourly intervals in one day.

Nov. 7th. General state is better; appetite better. Nightmares still occur, though less frequently.

Nov. 21st. No change.

Nat. Mur. 10M. Three doses, four hourly intervals in one day.

Dec. 10th. No nightmares. Looking noticeably better.

Jan. 17th. General health good; appetite good. No nightmares; no depression.

Feb. 15th. Mental state normal. No nightmares; no depression. General health decidedly better. Appetite good and gaining weight.

In Jahr's *Symptom Codex* we find under *Nat-Mur.* sleep symptoms 'Frightful dreams of murder, fire'. 'He rises at night from anxious dreams, and walks about the room.' 'Talking while asleep and restless night'. 'Moaning while asleep.'

Hahnemann's great work *The Chronic Diseases*, presents the same symptoms, as also does Allen's *Encyclopaedia of Pure Materia Medica.*

As a possible causative factor in the case presented, is the fact, that the girl's mother divorced her first husband, the father of the girl, and then married a second time. The circumstances appeared to affect the child deeply and aroused in her an attitude of partially suppressed resentment toward her mother. Psychic shock more often requires *Ignatia* in the beginning, followed by *Nat. mur.* later on.

Miss D., age 32 years, has been under drug treatment for many months on account of chronic tonsillitis and also the fact that it takes several hours for her to get to sleep. For the last eight years she has been taking hypnotics, i.e. prior to throat symptoms developing. Had heard how much a friend has been benefited by Homoeopathic constitutional treatment and now seeks assistance. Casually, during an otherwise rambling account, the patient remarked that for the last few years she could not go to a concert and could not bear to make music herself, as she was intensely affected there by (excited and then tired, or unable to get to sleep). Thereupon *Nat-carb* 30 was given every second evening for one week. This remedy has, in its proving, the symptom *Aggravation through music*. The result was remarkable. The long standing tonsillitis cleared up and the patient has been able to sleep well at night for the last three years.

Mr. B.D., a middle aged man of robust health, but sedentary occupation, had been in the habit of taking small doses of bicarbonate of soda for minor stomach symptoms. On one occasion he inadvertently took washing soda by mistake; this was followed by some epigastric burning and distress and later by hiccough, which persisted in spite of cathartics and other measures resorted to by his local doctor. After two days of this persistent singultus (Hiccough), he came for advice accompanied by a relative who had some years previously benefitted by Homoeopathy. This is what presented: almost constant hiccough, for two days past. Abuse of cathartics. Frequent inclination for stool, irritable state of the rectum (not surprising). Hiccough wakes him at 3 a.m. and is certainly very much worse at this hour. I gave him a few powders of *Nux. vom* 30, with instructions to take one every two hours. After the second powder the hiccough ceased, never to return.

Mrs. A.M., aged 38 years, mother of one child aged fourteen. No other pregnancies. For over a year under orthodox treatment. Has been advised to have either an ovarian operation or to be placed in a sanitorium. She was taken to her mother's home.

At last menstrual period, or just preceding the period she would become extremely violent, jumping out of bed and breaking ornaments, windows, and attempting to break furniture. Would scream, laugh, and make grotesque faces when spoken to. All this mental state would subside as soon as the flow was established. This condition lasting from a few hours to a day. At the appearance of the menstrual flow, although the mental symptoms abated she would be completely prostrated and would remain in bed nearly the whole time. She was heavily drugged when her mother finally brought her to me and I was able to understand little she had to say. I telephoned her mother the following day and asked her if she would come to see me without the patient. A sensible, clear thinking woman, she was able to give a most accurate account of her daughter's symptoms, which were many, but a flood of light was thrown on the case when she said 'I always know when these attacks are coming, because she always has looseness of bowels before the attack'. This was the KEY to the situation. I gave her *Bovista* 200 for two days. There was no return of the hysteria or mania, and four years later remains in excellent health.

Mrs. E.S., age 54 years, a somewhat sensitive anaemic, nervous lady, came under treatment in April 1964. She had been suffering for several weeks with a violent facial neuralgia involving the upper middle branches of the fifth nerve on the left side, the seat of the pain being over the left eye and in the left cheek. The patient described the pain as burning and sticking. Although during the day she was not wholly free from pain the acme of its intensity was about 11 p.m., and it was so violent then that even if she was already asleep she would have to spring out of bed on account of it, as also of the palpitation and anxiety accompanying it, all of which lasted some hours. A few powders of *Ars-Alb* 30 were prepared and patient instructed to take three powders, one at four hourly intervals and to have finished them by 8 p.m. that evening. Soon after taking the last powder all pain ceased and rest, quiet and sleep came to her.

Mrs. C.R.B., age 42 years, for years had been martyr to sick headaches. Almost without exception she would have an attack every time she went from home. Let her go to friends, go shopping take a day's visit, entertain company at home, or in fact do anything which called for a little extra or unusual exertion on her part, and the headache was sure to follow. The pain was located in the forehead, there was blurring of vision, inability to sit up or walk about, and great nausea attended by vomiting. The remedy in the 12th potency was sent to her with directions to take one dose when the first symptom of headache was felt. Repeat the dose every thirty minutes, until three doses were taken. Then stop and await results.

For years, this lady had seldom missed an attack of sick headache once a week and frequently several times a week.

I was delighted to hear at the end of one month, that every attack had been warded off by a few doses of *Epiphegus* 12.

This patient no longer has occasion to take any medicine at all, and it is now over two years since her last headache.

Mr. C.L., age 77 years, a slight, wiry, somewhat irritable man came to my rooms late one forenoon, he was an old patient of mine and had been keeping in good health over the past three years and had not had occasion to visit me, but now presented with a very bad cough which had continued for over a week, during which time he could not sleep, and had become weak, even staggering. As his general symptoms — they were well marked — not the cough — called for *Nux-Vom.*, I gave him one dose of *Nux.* 30. After 2 p.m. he felt calm and quiet. He slept all night without waking, and felt refreshed and stronger; cough much looser, expectoration free, pain entirely absent. Felt so much better he telephoned me to let me know, and in another 48 hours he was completely well.

Miss N.E., age 50 years, a finely bred sensitive woman suffering with paranoia was brought to me by her brother. She felt she had been jilted by a relative's poor judgement. She threw things at staff, kicked doors, struck different members of the family.

I found that the peculiar symptoms, the generals and particulars — the totality — pointed to *Nat. Mur.* This I gave, commencing with the 10M. I gave her six doses in a little over two years, twice on the ten thousandth plane, twice on the fifty-thousandth and twice on the hundred-thousandth plane, and at long intervals. Carefully checking and reviewing the case before each new prescription was made. The last time I saw her was at one of her sister's receptions. She was helping to entertain the guests, happy herself, and able to give happiness to others.

Mrs. P.B., age 48 years, dark hair, dark skin, brown eyes, with an inherited gouty constitution, had different abdominal complaints since her marriage with an unsympathetic husband. The most severe trouble was a painful affection of the spleen which dated back to her contracting malaria in the middle east. It was an almost constant digging, gnawing pain which deprived her of all desire for food and even of living. At the same time she was tormented by obstinate constipation and urinary disturbance. She walks bent forwards and with some insecurity. I gave *Ceanothus* 3. 1 drop every three hours in a teaspoonful of water. Within 7 days there was a notable improvement, and in another 7 days complete cessation of the splenic pains, as also of the other troubles. She was able to walk upright, her desire for life had returned, and she looked ten years younger.

Miss A.P., age 15 years. Two years ago, while at a picnic, sprained her ankle and otherwise badly hurt her foot. The foot was X-rayed which showed no bones fractured. She recovered sufficiently to be able to walk about as usual, but could never remain on her feet for any length of time nor walk any distance without her foot swelling and becoming exceedingly painful, and this condition seemed to grow worse rather than better. *Symphytum* ∅ was applied locally and *Symphytum* 30 given internally. The result was that very soon the pain ceased, for the first time in two years the foot was absolutely free from swelling, and today is as strong as ever, and the longest walks produce not the slightest discomfort.

Mr. B.M. aged 38 years, presented with migraine of twenty years standing, the attacks lasting from three days to three weeks. So severe, *'hardly knows what to do'*. Head very tender, cannot bear being touched, and the sickness which accompanies these awful attacks, lasting ten hours with vomiting every fifteen minutes. Cannot eat, therefore very weak. Feels very well just before an attack, a phenomenon not infrequent in the migraine syndrome, and knows the attack is coming.

Good family history; also general history good. Burrows head in pillow, no relief from anything. Feels as if suffocated if tries a little milk, which greatly aggravates the head pain. Normally is not very fond of milk, but tries it to sooth his stomach between the retching, which causes him so much agony. Does not like fat. Cannot understand why he gets so sleepy about 8 p.m. Large shiny bald patches on scalp diagnosed as Alopecia areata. Generally patient feels *'off-colour'*, i.e. generally less well, in hot weather, also before thunderstorms and after sleep.

Nat. mur 30 — three doses four hours apart, given.

Three weeks later. Not been laid up with his headache for the past three weeks; has not been sick, but generally still not feeling well. Has had a cold and is heavy and dull.

April. One attack threatened but passed off. When they came on before, they always laid him up for a week. He feels stronger, brighter, more heart for things. Sleep less heavy. Hair the same.

May 7th. Felt nauseated on the 3rd inst., but was not sick; only headache, same character.

Nat. mur 30 × 2 × 4 four hours apart.

July. Has been on holiday and not attended for nearly 8 weeks. Had four attacks since here, two bad. Same character.

Bry 30. Four powders three-hourly.

August. Headache much better but still 'in the background'.

Nat. mur 200 three doses four hours apart.

Sept. Not had an attack since last visit, despite anxious time at his business. Feels very well.

Nov. Not had a migraine for two months! Feels very much better in himself too.

Jan. No suggestion of migraine attack. Cannot believe it. Hair regrown. Discharged.

Mrs. M.M.G. age 39 years. Asthma since three years of age, following severe whooping cough. Has tried many treatments. Frequently spends three or four days of the week in bed. Very nervous and sensitive to noise. Hurrying or physical exertion, if prolonged, will bring on a sudden attack and her doctor has to give adrenalin. Likes warm room and warm clothing but breathing becomes difficult if room is too warm. Cigarette smoke also aggravates. Feet always cold. Chilly person generally and asthma is also aggravated in cold air. Appetite poor. *Drosera* 200 brought about the most amazing change in this patient and although two other remedies were later indicated and played an important part in her recovery programme neither of them acted so dramatically as *Drosera*.

Mrs. A.T.P. aged 45 years. The most obstinate menstrual headaches for the past eight years. Has tried '*everything*'. Much depression. Apprehensive and changeable moods. One day feels fine, another day wretched. Tired; restless; cannot settle down to her duties. Feels generally less well in damp weather. Neuralgia in short paroxysms, in various places. Rheumatism, periodic, in long muscles. Head dull and confused much of the time and frequent sensation of band around the forehead. Headache most mornings, leaving later in the day. Intense pain during and after menstrual period. Begins late afternoon or wakens her between 2 and 4 a.m. Commences in temples, extending over entire head, and into teeth and jaw. Steady intense pain, throbbing when worst. Worse when lying down; from motion, light and noise, and is accompanied by intense restlessness. Nausea which is sometimes ameliorated by vomiting. Chilliness with perspiration. There is marked soreness in occiput and nape of neck after headache also the scalp is very sensitive. Heavy sleep, at times and often preceding the headache. Has fainted during the intense head pain. Likes to be out in the cool open air. *Nat. m.*, and then *Phos.*, were given with great relief from both remedies but they failed to hold for more than a few months. This told its own tale and led me to select *Tub-bov* 200 and later 1M. Since beginning with the new remedy, over a period of 10 months, her general health has improved in a most remarkable way and the awful headaches are a thing of the past.

Mrs. O.D. age 52 years. Presented with head and eye symptoms and blood pressure of 180/120. History of acute mania, three years previously, excessive nervousness has continued. Heart rapid and painful action and is greatly aggravated by any nervous shock or excitement and from thinking of disagreeable things. Unhappy, much mental depression, often with suicidal thoughts. Very dizzy on looking down also when walking and with a tendency to drop things. Heat flushes are most distressing.

Sepia 30 given. Three weeks later 'feeling better', blood pressure 170/105.

One month later, blood pressure 140/80.

The patient is a happy, cheerful, enthusiastic women. All symptoms gone.

Miss H. age 30 years, has been sick for many years, and very poorly for some months. She now seeks Homoeopathic treatment and wants relief from a severe, agonizing headache. The pain is described as a pressure, or *crushing pain* on vertex, going to occiput like a weight or heavy wedge. At times is verging on delirious from the pain, and rolls head from side to side and thinks the pain is a little easier by pressing head back into pillow. Her eyes are very sensitive to light and the roof of mouth is swollen, sore and itching; feels like tearing it out with her finger nails and every tooth pains up into her head. Very thirsty, wants to drink all the time, but there is vomiting of food and water as soon as taken and the vomit is bitter, setting her teeth on edge. Says she aches all over and has cramping pains in legs, calves, feet and toes. Has had much grief and sorrow in her young life.

I have her *Phos-ac*. C.M. and general guidance regarding these terrible head pains.

One week later: Reported '*much better generally*'.

Another three weeks went by when patient presented herself at my rooms. The pain had begun yesterday afternoon and although not nearly so badly as when she first sought treatment, she was frightened the excrutiating pains would return.

Phos.ac. C.M. three doses were given at four hourly intervals.

One week later: Reported 'the pain just disappeared'.

Mr F.M.I. aged 48 years. Tall, fair, lean, bad head wounds during war service. Has had 'indigestion' for the last eight years; is a heavy eater, and after a hearty meal has a heavy sensation in stomach. His head began to trouble him three years ago. Has heard of the advantages of Homoeopathic medication and now seeks assistance.

In the right parietal region there is numbness, a gnawing sensation and neuralgic pains at times. Tenderness in the occipital region, and in the right temple there is a feeling as if the blood did not circulate properly: there is numbness and slight itching, and he rubs the temple and side of the head vigorously to get relief. The neuralgic pains are noticeable after overeating.

He gets muddled from reading, and being in law and a conscientious worker, he is a hard reader, and lately has had to avoid everything but his own work, as he would be quite incapable after a few days reading. His concentration is remarkable and evidently exhaustive. He says mental exertion pulls him right down and he gets irritable, so that he does not want to talk to anyone; says he is physically and mentally exhausted.

He always feels better from physical exertion, especially walking in the sunshine, and is very fond of the open air. Likes the warm weather of summer, likes cold weather also. Has never had the same feeling in the head since being wounded in 1941 and feels that if the right side of the head were well he would be all right.

Has a peculiar sore sensation about the heart at times, as if it were being pulled out. The right side of the hard palate feels as if being eaten away; a gnawing feeling for more than a year. Has some numbness in the right hand and foot and slighter in the corresponding arm and leg, and this is relieved by exercise. Drinking liquids at meals causes pain at the base of the brain. Has a craving occasionally for sugar and thinks he feels better after eating some. Has a clear watery discharge from right nostril and right eye at times; may come twice a week or three or four days in succession, with an interval of a week or ten days.

On January 4th, 1963 I gave him *Aurum-met* 10m. and he began to improve in a few weeks.

In the August 1963 when he was discharged he said he had as good a stomach as when he was 21, his *indigestion* being a thing of the past.

He had done much reading, besides his regular law work and his head did not get muddled, said it was 'first rate' and not influenced by mental exertion as formerly. His weight in January was 135 lbs. and in August 155 lbs. The stomach symptoms of eight years standing and the head symptoms completely gone and patient stated he did not know when he had enjoyed such good health.

The next is a short case to illustrate the speed with which Homoeopathic medicines work in acute illness.

Mr. J.F.M. age 55 years.

Dec. 8th. Staggered into my rooms, extremely ill with influenza.

How he ever made the journal I will never understand.

There was complete loss of strength.

No thirst at all.

A sore, tired ache, all over.

Feels very ill.

Apathetic condition; wants to be quiet; wants to close eyes yet no photophobia.

Soft palate swollen and red about the throat.

Much tough, stringy mucus, gagging but no nausea.

White coated tongue bearing imprint of teeth.

Uring highly coloured and scanty.

No stool for three days.

Dryness of the lips.

Coldness of the knees.

Sense of chilliness and heat at the same time.

Chin-ars. 1M. three doses given, to be taken at two hourly intervals.

Sent home in a taxi.

Dec. 9th. Entirely well today. Bowels moved yesterday evening. Appetite returned and feels generally well.

A fine cure.

Mr B — age 40, a case of nervous exhaustion.

A heavy, strong looking man; habits regular and correct; florid, healthy in appearance.

Symptoms:— Very weak; a short walk exhausts him and brings on a pain extending from the neck to the top of the head. He has occasional palpitation with fulness and pain in head. Sleeps very little, an hour or two on going to bed, then lies awake most of the night. Cold sweat on legs and thighs at night. Flushes of heat with redness of face from slight exercise. Pulsation felt in region of stomach. Is very apprehensive, fears a stroke and heart disease. If he lay down in the day time the upper side of body broke out in profuse perspiration. On turning to that the perspiration disappeared from it and appeared on the other side.

Benzinum 30 was administered with immediate improvement, and finally, complete cure.

Mrs. S.B. — age 52 years. Came to be treated for rheumatism(?).

Has for many months an aggravating pain in lower back, has tried several treatments but now the pains are getting worse and have extended gradually down the back on the left thigh and leg, are very severe now, shooting downward, lightning like, and produce cramping pains in the calf. They are accompanied with a sticking, pressing, burning pain in the stomach; nausea and vomiting, which is worse after eating or drinking coffee or water. Water is vomited immediately after drinking, and, though she is very thirsty, because of the vomiting, she drinks little, yet often. She has no appetite, the smell or sight of food nauseates. Eating or drinking increases the burning in stomach; pains in lumbar region are aggravated by misstep. She is restless, must walk about, and the pains in the leg are relieved from walking and warmth. She looks pale and emaciated and feels worse in general about 1 a.m. The pain in back is much worse on rising from a chair.

She received *Cocculus Indicus* 200, a powder to be dissolved in six teaspoons of water, to take one teaspoon every two hours.

She improved with the first dose, continued to do so slowly but steadily and one week later pronounced herself cured.

Mrs. C.D. age 45 years, had been seen by several specialists over a period of eighteen months before she was brought to me by a relation who had recently benefited by my treatment. Poor Mrs. D. could not face the ordeal of a journey, even with her dearest friends, she could not travel by train or bus, or go to any place of entertainment — fear of crowds, fear of being closed in was her unfortunate condition of mind. She could not go out in the dark or be alone by day. She could not cross a street or walk along a busy thoroughfare, and many other idiosyncrasies held her in bondage.

She was full of fears, fear of people; dogs; the dark; men; closed places; high buildings and high places. If she attempted to cross a road, she would become transfixed halfway across, sink down to a crumpled heap and tremble with fear until someone came to her assistance and led her to the other side. If she went out with her husband or friend and came into a busy place she would stop suddenly and tremble — she could not go forward or backwards until the trembling passed off and then she would be giddy and appear like an intoxicated person, flushed and dazed. Periodically at night she would wake up in a fright, which ended in a bout of weeping and sobbing, then a coma-like snoring condition for the remainder of the night.

On the physical side she was a thyrotoxic case. Suffered from flatulent dyspepsia also abnormal menstrual periods. T.B. glands had been removed from her neck when she was a child. She had been the usual round of medical men but they had been unable to help her and fortunately her husband, a pharmacist, had prevented her from taking some of the pernicious drugs which had been prescribed. She was so complete a nervous case: Hysteria, Irritability, Hypersensitive, Hypochondriacal, Neurasthenic; a case so full of trouble that one hardly knew where to begin.

The bulging eyes were shouting for attention, the scars at the side of her neck, the flushed face and throbbing carotids; the anxiety and trembling; the hard breathing, like a moan; the sensation of a crawling from the right foot to the face and head, ending in a facial spasm and a sensation as if the hair was standing on end; the almost constant belching and water-brash — Oh! my, what a mess! Am I writing about one patient? Yes, that was Mrs. D., two years ago, when as a last resort she was brought to me for help.

Tub.bov., Arg.Nit., and the occasional dose of *Aconite* 200 for some acute exacerbation, worked miracles for this ill woman.

It was an extreme case and not accomplished without hard work and some disappointments, but many successes also to be proud of and thankful for. Slowly but surely health returned to this patient and the days of torture gradually changed to days of happiness and conscious delight.

Miss N. — age 22 years consulted me because of an unsightly eruption on the face and on the lips which had resisted the efforts of several dermatologists. At first glance I realised there was something quite wrong with this patient, apart from the local skin lesion. Miss N. was 22 years old but she looked more than 30. She was very tall, a skeleton covered with a dead-looking yellow, earthy skin; she lived largely on hot, strong tea, fried food, puddings, potatoes and condiments of every kind.

Careful questioning revealed that prior to the skin eruption, the patient was stung on the left ankle by an insect. 'The ankle and foot swelled prodigiously and then the leg and the right leg went similarly. My legs were immovable, paralysed, and this went on for several weeks.'

The insect sting had, as happens occasionally, produced blood poisoning — I have seen an apparently incurable paralysis of several years standing caused by insect stings, which I was fortunate enough to cure with *Apis* and *Ledum*, and this was a similar case. This girl was going to pieces owing to the latent low grade blood poisoning; she had lost a good deal of weight and now this unsightly facial eruption had developed. Modern medicine often overlooks the obvious. She rapidly improved under *Apis* 30 and later on *Sulph.* 200, put on weight and looked ten years younger after a few months treatment.

These medicines counteracted the poisons from the insect sting which had caused the trouble, and together with the adjustments I had made in her faulty eating habits, built up her constitution, resulting in renewed health and vigour.

Mr. R.N.L. — age 34 years. Asthma for past 7 years. Has seen a number of specialists and received a corresponding variety of advice and treatment.

He felt the cold considerably and was greatly distressed by the paroxysms of asthma which occurred most evenings, particularly if he was not mentally occupied. The attacks were often aggravated by change of weather; worse from damp air, and when he was mentally depressed, although he suffered no anxiety during the attacks. His general health prior to the commencement of the asthma, had always been good, and the past history revealed nothing that could account for this deviation from his previous healthy state. Careful consideration of the above symptoms revealed indications for *Phos.* 30, which cured this man in nine months, he gained twelve pounds in weight and now, five years later, there has never been the slightest suggestion of asthma.

Mr. P.R. aged 44 years. A strong muscular man, whilst moving things in the store room at home received a severe bruise in the lower left chest from the corner of a falling trunk. He was examined by a surgeon friend, sent for X-ray, where no ribs were found to be broken.

Several days later pain commenced in his chest, it had kept him awake for two nights and he had been groaning with the pain. This pain was worse from any motion of the body or any jarring or touch in the bruised region. He came to see me at 11 a.m. on a Wednesday one week after the accident. The remedy was easy to see and I gave him one dose of *Arnica* 1m and two more to be taken home and used if necessary with instructions to let me know how he responded. In three days he returned eager to know what magic was in the medicine. He said he could walk erect before he had reached home, could move with much less pain, could touch the sore chest and even bear some pressure. He had slept all that night, felt incredibly better next morning, and returned to his business that same day. He needed no more medicine.

Mrs. A.D.M., aged 72 years. An apprehensive, nervous little lady, she had been subject to severe attacks of indigestion for many years and when very acute she had sometimes fainted. In July 1963 she had the worst attack she had ever experienced. Her daughter, a patient of mine, asked me to call on her mother, and living close by I saw her at 6 p.m. that evening. She was throwing herself about in bed, obviously in great pain, declaring that she was dying, and looking as if she might at any moment. Her face was pale, pinched, bluish, cold, with an anguished expression. Severe pain in stomach and abdomen and oppression of chest over area of the heart. Gasping for breath. Violent nausea with frequent vomiting. Copious diarrhoea of intensely foul odour; pulse quick and weak.

I quickly dissolved a powder of *Ars. Alb.* 1m. in a wine glass of water and three teaspoons were given, each at five minute intervals.

The pain started to improve after the second dose and ceased after the third. No more vomiting, no more diarrhoea.

When the pain had ceased she was prostrated, too weak to move or talk; pulse was thready and uncertain. Two hours later, no return of pain, diarrhoea, etc., but pulse still thready. One dose of *Ars-Alb* 1m., was placed on her tongue and in a few minutes the pulse was steady and she soon slept.

Recovery was excellent with no return of the trouble.

Miss C.G. aged 49 years. A history of gall stone colic for past six years, paroxysms occurring at intervals of one to three months. Although she had received various treatments, the paroxysms were increasing in both frequency and intensity. The following symptoms were given a few days after an acute attack:—

April 4th — The pain so intense it occasions unconsciousness. *Unbearable; it appears that she cannot endure it; that it would drive her insane.* Begins always in the evening, continuing until midnight. Preceded by intense pressure in 'pit of stomach', as if from a stone. *Irritable; cross; does not want to be disturbed.* Mouth bitter taste, much worse in the mornings. Desires acid fruits, citrus etc. Aversion to coffee. Eructations sour; odour of spoiled eggs; painful. Vomiting of green, sour, bitter mucus. Stitching pains in liver; sensation of fullness 'as if liver is swollen'. Hypochondria, sensitive to pressure, even of clothes. Menstrual period still with her, too early and profuse, with dark clots. Before period commences has a cutting pain from back to front also bearing down pains extending to thighs. Backache at night, the muscles feel bruised. Arms 'go to sleep' at night; pains awaken her. All her pains are aggravated by heat and are worse in the evening to midnight. *Cham* 1M — 3 doses at four hourly intervals were given.

Two weeks later.

All symptoms relieved. More cheerful than has felt for months.

Three weeks later.

All symptoms relieved.

Last menstrual period normal as to time and quantity, no clotting. Pain slight.

Hypochondria soreness entirely absent.

Back pain absent.

To report again in a month.

June. Says her general health is better than for seven years.

August. No symptoms remain, 'feels marvellous'.

In January of the following year her husband came to consult me and I had the opportunity of meeting my patient again, at the same time to learn there had been no recurrence and her good health continued.

Mrs. S.M. age 36 years. Eczema of many years duration.

The eruption over both shins almost reaching to knees. She had been troubled with dry scaly eruption in this area which became decidedly worse every Spring and Autumn. The eruption was painful, burning, itching and now oozing watery fluid. The itching became intensified when the affected areas were uncovered and was soothed by cold applications. Almost lame from the pain and swelling and with some oedema of both legs and the legs were always cold. Has frequent headaches which commence in the nape of the neck and extend up over the head; nose bleeds often accompany these headaches and the forehead feels icy cold. Menstrual period is regular but has much cramping pain. Strong smells nauseate. Frequent heat flushes (not menopausal) followed by perspiration, and then shivering. Appetite was poor and fatty foods disagreed. Continually sighing and has palpitation when excited or nervous, which is sometimes aggravated by lying on the left side. Palms perspire and feet used to when she was younger, with an offensive perspiration. Is uncomfortable in a warm room but open air makes her chilly. Likes plenty of covers on her bed.

March 3rd — Commenced treatment with *Sil*. 200 — unit dose.

March 31st — Feeling very much better. Less pain in eruption. Swelling of legs subsiding.

April 28th — Slight headache for a week. Began in nape of neck and travelled to forehead. Forehead cold and applied warmth comforting. *Skin eruption healing.*

May 26th — Foot sweat of childhood has returned (on the road to extinction) profuse and with offensive odour. *Skin eruption entirely healed.*

June 30th — No sight of where eruption had been. No pain with menstrual period. No headaches at all. No foot perspiration. Patient enjoying new found health.

Mrs. E.L. age 30 years, married, two children.

Metrorrhagia (irregular haemorrhage from the uterus). Trouble has now existed for six years, during which she has received much treatment including curettage etc., etc. Is flowing all the time. Patient weak and anaemic from the continuous drain on her system. Menstruation early, ten days before time and duration of ten days — bright in colour, profuse, accompanied by headache and bearing down sensations.

Aversion to much covering, wants to be cool, cannot stand a warm room. Sensation as though pins and needles were pricking her feet, worse when standing or walking; also some numbness of feet. Flow aggravated by any physical exertion, and during flow is very weak. Dragging down sensation is felt from umbilicus. *Secale* 200 was given on June 8th.

July 2nd — Last menstrual period lasted 7 days; were profuse the first two days, dark and clotted. Bearing down pains and backache.

July 30th — Feeling better in herself. Numbness of feet much better.

August 27th — Last period, duration 6 days and were normal in appearance and quantity.

Some treatment for her constitutional condition followed, and soon the general debility was replaced by radiant health, with the increased well being that accompanies it.

Rev. X. A clergyman age 45 years. Had been working extremely hard and under considerable emotional strain for some time. Result? Nervous collapse! He could not sleep, even with sleeping tablets prescribed by his doctor; was emaciated and so weak that he could scarcely speak and could walk about the house only with great difficulty. The tongue was heavily coated, appetite gone. He suffered from pains running up the back and into the head, was utterly depressed and helpless. The reflexes were exaggerated. He was extremely nervous and all his troubles were aggravated by noise.

Nux vom. made a new man of him in eight weeks.

RHEUMATISM AND ARTHRITIS in their various forms are crippling complains which have so often defeated the best efforts of orthodox medicine and whilst it would be inaccurate to suggest that Homoeopathy has found the complete answer to them, it has, nevertheless, been my experience that a very high percentage of chronic cases of rheumatism can be cleared up and many cases of arthritis with due regard to the extent of the pathology, can be greatly helped.

Mrs. E.T., age 68 was brought to my rooms by car in March, 1964 and with great difficulty, much pain and shuffling gait made her way to the chair from which she related to me a history of rheumatoid arthritis of the hands with ulnar deviation, etc. dating back to 1940 but during the past few years both the knee joints had become involved.

The knees were very painful in the morning on rising with agonising pain at times when moving about and the knee joints felt as though they were '*grinding together*', only free from pain when completely still — sensitive to draughts and frosty weather, aspirins upset her stomach and fatty food disagreed. Being a sensitive lady, she was, quite naturally, most depressed by her condition.

The management of this case, in which both rheumatoid and osteoarthritis were present, improvement of the patient and observing the action of carefully spaced doses of her constitutional remedy has afforded me much pleasure, but none so great as when, nine months from commencing treatment, this lady after a journey which entailed boarding five different buses and a train journey to London, *completely alone and unaided*, walked into my rooms.

Mr. T.F.S. aged 61 years, a brilliant athlete when a young man and had been capped for England, he was still a fine figure of a man and did not look his age, but for the past seven years had suffered from '*chronic rheumatism of the joints*'; it disappears for several days at a time only to come flooding back with all its old intensity — has tried many treatments unsuccessfully.

Examination revealed the joints to be swollen and the pains to be of a stinging, tearing character. The tearing pains compelled the patient to move, on which the pains extended down the limbs and accompanied at times with jerking of the muscles. The pains were usually worse from warmth, worse in the evening and on beginning to move though eventually eased a little by moving slowly from one room to another.

The indications suggested Chronic Infective Arthritis and I suspected a focus of infection somewhere but the symptom totality pointed to *Pulsatilla which cured this patient in four months* and now five years have passed and the patient continues in robust health.

THE MENOPAUSE or change of life, is the epoch at which the reproductive activity of the female undergoes involution and the menses, which are the sign of that activity, cease. This may take place in three ways:— (a) the menses may cease gradually, appearing at gradually lengthening intervals until finally they stop altogether; (b) they may cease quite suddenly; (c) there may be a series of haemorrhages.

When menstruation ceases at the normal age of the menopause, in a *perfectly healthy woman*, this process takes place with no disturbance of her normal life. The fact there is so much attendant phenomena at the menopause is, to me, more indicative of patients requiring *constitutional treatment to regulate their general health*, than it is solely characteristic of the menopause.

The following cases will help to illustrate this:

Mrs. L.A. — age 46 years, had been ill for about two years. Complained of severe headaches, distressing heat flushes, a dreadful faint feeling, besides other ailments and at times wished she could die.

Suffered much from acidity of the stomach for many years past — before entering the change — often with cramping pains. When the acidity was bad she vomited and the acrid fluid made her teeth feel so sharp that it was intolerable for her tongue to touch them. Her doctor had given antacids and for the flushes had given oestrogen (sex hormones) which thoroughly disagreed with her and had to be discontinued. Now, as a last hope she turned to Homoeopathy.

Sepia in ascending potencies plus a dose of *Psorinum* when the symtoms changed to indicate it and back to *Sepia* again a month or so later completely transformed this ailing woman together with absolute disappearance of the symptoms of the change.

In short, a prescription based on the deranged health of the patient which existed prior to the menopause, restored her health and wiped out all the symptoms, *including those of the menopausal syndrome.*

Mrs. A.P.T., age 53 years, of frail appearance. Menopause commenced three years ago with the familiar pattern of hot flushes and much nervous phenomena, insomnia, irritability, depression, etc. Previous history of post nasal and laryngeal catarrh for many years, much stomach disturbances, rheumatism, occasional asthmatic respiration; an extremely chilly patient, very sensitive to draughts, much anxiety and fear in her make up and many of her symptoms worse during the first few hours after midnight.

Kali-Ars. cured.

All symptoms including the intractable catarrh which dated back to childhood, completely cured, *plus those of the menopause.*

To every reader I take this opportunity to stress that all irregular uterine bleeding, before, during or after the change must *always be investigated by careful and thorough gynaecological examination and not simply attributed to the change of life.*

Miss — age 50 years, Matron of a large institution had received antibiotic therapy for an abscess in the ear and although the acute condition had responded to treatment the ear continued to discharge and the patient was extremely debilitated. She had written to me three months previously and I had explained that it was impossible to prescribe without seeing her and now, as other treatment had failed to help her she reported for examination and treatment.

Knowing that there must be a constitutional defect behind her illness, and that to treat successfully, the remedy must be based on the totality of her symptoms, I elicited an account of her various other ailments, too long to report here, and learnt that her doctor had three times sent her to bed, and she felt as though her vitality and strength were leaving her.

Her symptoms clearly indicated *Lycopodium* which I gave her in the 30th potency at the beginning of June, her progress then was marvellous and on the 4th July she was able to resume her duties. This lady has sent me many patients and some she has brought to me in person; I have, therefore, had the opportunity of observing that *her health was permanently restored.*

Mr. T.F. — age 48 years. Tall and painfully thin, when this patient first came to see me the short journey from his London hotel to my rooms had utterly exhausted him. Though under fifty he looked seventy. The trouble began with attacks of dysentery during the war, which led up to violent and uncontrollable mucous discharges from the bowel, the mucous masses were often as large as the palm of the hand. He had consulted leading authorities who could only recommend rest and extreme care in diet. By this time he could barely walk a hundred yards without resting, had not eaten most vegetables for years, but lived entirely on milk, fish and white of chicken.

He also suffered from palpitations and restless, broken sleep; his mouth and palate were sore, his tongue furred, his skin excessively dry, a disagreeable tremor of the head, a milky urethral discharge, and emissions were a nightly occurrence.

After twelve weeks patient reported 'my bowels move properly each day, the motions are healthy and the discharge of mucus much less. There is no milky discharge from the urethra. No nocturnal emissions for nearly three weeks. My appetite is good and sleep sound. The tremor of the head also ceases for intervals. My skin looks healthier.'

At the end of six months there was indeed a striking change in this man. He looked bright and his eyes had a healthy appearance; he had put on weight and his mental depression was gone. He could eat meat, vegetables, and indeed, almost anything.

I kept this patient under observation for over five years and while he naturally experienced the usual fluctuations of health due to family worries, an attack of influenza, etc., *he never once relapsed into his old condition.*

Aloe Socotrina; Kali Bichromicum; and *Natrum Muriaticum* were the principal remedies employed in the cure of this patient.

Mrs. L.D., age 72 years, had been suffering for three or four years from serious attacks of jaundice; her doctor failing to give her relief advised operation but no mechanical obstruction was found.

She finally decided to try Homoeopathy. The case presented the usual features, and some unusual. There was a constant but variable jaundice; yellow discoloration, becoming a deep brown during the attacks. The acute attacks were seldom less than one a week, often every few days; they came on generally in the forenoon and lasted all day; a severe chill felt first and most in the back requiring an electric blanket plus all the extra blankets that could be piled on; marked thirst during the chill and delirium all day; finally sweat during the evening with relief. The remedy was clearly indicated and its administration gave almost immediate relief, reducing the attacks to one a month, but slight indiscretions of diet continued to bring them on, though with greatly lessened severity.

The remedy was *Capsicum* 1M. Three months after beginning

treatment, I gave her *Sulph* 200 to reach the underlying psoric miasm, a short reaction followed and I was telephoned for by an anxious member of the family; on seeing the patient my advice to the family was simply *'wait and see'* — within a few days she started to pick up and recovery was completely uneventful. Over two years have passed without any return of the jaundice, her skin remains nice and pink and instead of being thin and scraggy as before, she is now plump like a young person and as sprightly and gay as a woman many years her junior. It is reasonably safe to consider this case cured.

Mr. A.L.G. age 44 years had for three years a large irritating patch on his leg, he had shown it to his doctor friend who immediately diagnosed it as psoriasis — various treatments were tried but none proved successful. He consulted me in April 1958 and the case outline was certainly very meagre; perfect health except for the skin trouble; fond of meat, eggs, salt and sweets; history of scabies three times during war service in the army. *Sulph* 200 wrought a complete cure within six weeks, so complete and so remarkable that he again showed his leg to his doctor friend, who was very much at a loss to account for it but assured him he was exceedingly fortunate, with which I heartily concur, as psoriasis can prove most stubborn before finally surrendering to treatment.

Mr. M.J.T. age 56 years, another case of psoriasis; in perfect health, not a symptom to be had, but fortunately a clear history. It seems the trouble had been very marked in his childhood, and had at that time been cured or suppressed with Fowlers Solution in material doses. It presented no difficulty at all to administer *Kali Arsenicum* 10M, and that single exhibition of the remedy removed it entirely in a short time and the case itself serving as a classical example of the importance of past history.

Early in May 1960 I was called in on a case reported to be chronic rheumatoid arthritis. I found the patient, a lady of 78 years of age, in bed, hands and feet swollen and patient in much pain. In addition, the previous night she had a slight stroke of paralysis, on left side, left arm and hand, left leg and foot almost helpless, with the left side of face slightly drawn to the left side. She was almost speechless, articulation very difficult and memory severely impaired.

I learned that the arthritis was of eighteen months duration, had received steroid therapy to which she at first responded but relapsed badly after a few months. She had complained of severe pains in her face which were considerably relieved by warm compresses.

The only turning point in the history of this patient, who had previously enjoyed good health, was an attack of shingles two months prior to the onset of the rheumatoid arthritis, her face had been badly affected and convalescence extremely slow, in fact had barely recovered when struck down by the arthritis.

The laboratory report gave the following:

Blood — uric acid 8.6.

Haemoglobin 53.

Leucocytes greatly in excess.

On questioning a relative, the additional feature of the patients pains being great aggravated when 'rain was about' came to light.

I gave a unit dose of *Rhus-Tox* 10m with the instruction that the patient be given no other medicine and another chemical analysis of the blood to be made in 14 days.

The next report showed:

Uric acid 3.3.

Haemoglobin 73.

The trace of albumin found in previous analysis was absent.

Pain considerably less and patient much better in herself generally.

I then gave *Urtica Urens* mother tincture 5 mins ex aq tid., to encourage elimination of uric acid, introduced vitamin therapy and other ancillary measures.

The patient continued to progress and during the warm days of July and August was strong enough to take occasional walks.

Two things are to be learnt from this case, (a) the ability of the highly attenuated remedy to influence the chemistry of the blood and (b) the invaluable lesson that instead of experimenting with unproved remedies in treating the sick, as some do, we ourselves should be encouraged to study more intensely the well proven remedies Homoeopathy has placed in our possession.

Mrs. M.J. age 42 years. Migraine with intense occipital and frontal pain, at irregular intervals for many years and often with nausea and vomiting. Headaches were aggravated by noise, draught, cold, anger, excitement and ameliorated by closing eyes, pressure of hand and hot applications. Has suffered from 'rheumatism on and off for years' with stiffness of all joints, pains were aggravated from motion, heat, cold and during the night.

She was apprehensive, mild, timid and fearful that something will happen to members of the family as well as a lot of general anxiety and fear in her make-up.

Her menstrual period was always early and with scanty flow. Alimentary symptoms only revealed that her stomach was disturbed in a vague way by certain foods at times, that she was fond of coffee but it made her sick. If anxious or depressed it was always worse in the evening.

After careful assessment of this case, symptom evaluation and repertorial study — *Causticum* 30 was selected and repeated when appropriately called for, over a period of six months — at the end of which, *no headaches at all, rheumatic pains completely gone, menstruation normal and patient enjoying robust health.*

This case is but another example of the importance of a strictly personal investigation of every patient, this patient had received treatment through the years from several good prescribers but somehow, the image of her personal remedy was missed — yet it was there, all the time, waiting to be uncovered.

Mrs. F. — aged 39, came to see me and gave the following history of her case:— For more than six months she has had frequent scanty, thin, brown stools, scanty as to quantity, expelled with force, with crampy pains in the abdomen before, during and after stool. Coldness over the whole body during stool, except in the face which is hot. Griping pains starting from both groins meet in the centre of the abdomen on a line with the groins; this pain is followed by a small evacuation, of the colour and consistency above mentioned, then a short interval, and then more pain and another stool. Tenesmus worse after stool, some also during the stool. Bearing down as if everything would protrude during stool; worse after stool. Debility after stool. The stools are always more frequent after lunch or tea; *never has any after breakfast.* Cramps in the calf of right leg after each stool. Thirst after the stool. During the whole of this time her appetite had continued good.

Three powders of *Trombidium* 200 were given, and she reported that within twenty-four hours there was a marked decrease in the number of stools, and much less pain, and within the next twenty-four hours the trouble had vanished.

Reasons for the selection of the remedy — The thin brown stools are found under *Lyc., Rheum., Rhod., Rumex* and *Trom.,* frequent scanty stools under *Canth., Caps., Cham., Coloc., Dulc., Merc., Merc-cor., Mez., Trom;* tenesmus during, principally under *Aloe, Ars., Bell., Colch. Iris., Kali-bich., Magn-c., Merc., Merc-cor., Nux-vom., Tabac.,* tenesmus after *Bell., Canth., Caps., Colch., Kali-bich., Magn-c., Merc., Merc-c., Rheum., Sulph., Tromb.* Stools more frequent after eating, the principal remedies are *Ars., Croton-tig., Lyc., Tromb.*

The remedies bearing the closest similarity to the remedy chosen, viz. Trombidium, are *Magn-c., Merc-cor.,* and *Merc-viv.,* but none of these have the *marked aggravation after eating*; and *the marked increase in the number of stools after lunch and tea, and not after breakfast.* The weakness after stool is found under *Ars.,*

Carb-veg., Con., Tromb and *Verat*; and all the other remedies which have any resemblance to the case are deficient in this condition.

Here was a case of over six months duration wiped out dramatically in forty-eight hours — *but here a reminder* — you will only do this kind of work with what I choose to call the *Absolute Similimum.*

Other remedies would have helped this patient, other remedies would finally have cured, but *only one* would cure in accordance with that laid down in the Organon, Para. 2.

'The highest ideal of cure is rapid, gentle and permanent restoration of the health, or removal and annihilation of the disease in its whole extent, in the shortest, most reliable and most harmless way', — and that was *Trombidium*, which, I submit, was the *Absolute Similimum.*

Miss X — age 42 years, was commonly supposed to be a hopeless case, after much professional and domestic medication. She was suffering from chronic gastritis with enormous abdominal distension, enlarged liver, alternate diarrhoea and constipation, and dysmenorrhoea (painful menstruation). Finally she was persuaded to 'try Homoeopathy'. I dissuaded a 'trial', and after some plain talk secured an unqualified enlistment.

Among her symptoms were these: Nausea after cold drinks; spitting up mouthfuls of undigested food, sour vomiting; incarcerated flatulence, relieved by heat; red sediment in urine. *Lycopodium* caused a material improvement *but did not cure*. Although she had become able to assist in various household affairs, she was not well. I watched her *very closely*, as in view of the many years the condition had been with her I was ever fearful of it taking on a malignant phase.

Then the following symptoms appeared: Cold, bluish, sweaty face, body and limbs: tongue yellow with red streak down the middle; restless sleep; full, hard pulse. *Veratrum viride* 200 in water, one dose each hour, for four doses brought about a dramatic change for the better. I prescribed rest and general care etc., as although pleased with her response to *Veratrum viride*, and encouraged by the overall improvement since commencing treatment, I knew she was not 'out of the wood'. Another month went by, during which she held the ground she had gained, but no further progress that I could determine. At this time she mentioned a new symptom of a heaviness on the chest and inability to breathe deeply enough. Bearing in mind the chronic nature of the case — the very definite improvement from *Lycopodium* — the beneficial, but more superficial action of *Veratrum viride*, the new symptom which had come forward under the beautiful action of these remedies, left me with the obvious choice of *Sulph* — a remedy complementary to and following well after *Lycopodium*, which had first set this lady on the path to recovery. Sulph 200, three doses at four hourly intervals completely cured this patient and one year later she writes to remind me of this and adds: 'Oh! I am thankful', . . . 'I am eating everything in sight'.

Mrs. E.R., age 38 years, gave me the following history:
At fourteen she began to menstruate and did so regularly until sixteen years of age, when it became rather erratic and the flow more profuse than usual. This lasted for several years when it settled down under Homoeopathic treatment, and no further trouble until 1963 when she presented herself with the following symptoms — Had been losing blood for over a year, has been curretted, but three weeks afterwards blood loss commenced again. The flow was bright red, no clots, thin and never changing in colour. Less when quiet at night; always worse when moving about, often quite profuse after any extra exertion. As a result of this flow, she was pale and weak but surprisingly enough, had not lost much weight, possibly owing to the fact that she had a good appetite and slept well. She could not tell why she was in this condition; what produced it was a mystery to her. She complained of intense weakness in lower bowel and lower part of spine.

I gave her *Erigeron* 30 three times daily for three days and the *flow stopped within five days*. Since when she has menstruated at regular intervals of twenty-eight days, the flow lasting three or four days and she reports herself '*well in every way*'.

Mrs. M.T., age 48 years, came to me complaining of loss of appetite and a severe indigestion with a great deal of flatulence in the stomach and bowels. She said she could not sleep well, was very depressed, and in fact did not care to keep on living. This woman had always enjoyed good health and was not of a nervous temperament. She was never hysterical and in fact showed no signs of grief to other people. She was keeping it all to herself. She was suffering from suppressed grief.

Some two or three years previously her husband was involved in a car accident in which his back was broken. He was operated on several times with no special benefit and after a great deal of suffering he died a few months previous to the time his widow came to see me.

Towards the end of the consultation I realised this woman was an *Ignatia* patient. I gave her *Ignatia* 30 three times daily for three days.

In two weeks she returned to see me saying that she felt a different person in every way. She felt more cheerful, slept well at night, had a good appetite and could eat anything she liked with no distress of any sort. And the cure was permanent.

Mr. C.M.J. age 60 years. Chief complaint, frequent, urgent desire to urinate. Urine passed in a feeble stream, and a sensation as though a drop remained in the urethra after urinating. Night frequency. No history of gonorrhoeal infection. Patient also complains of vertigo when rising up from a stooping position, occasional attacks of neuritis or sciatica, and lack of appetite. B.P. 100/68. Prostate slightly enlarged.

The miasm in this case was sycosis and the remedy for the patient was *Thuja* 200.

The result: in one month, no vertigo. B.P. 110/70. Urination better in every way. Over a period of two years, *Thuja* has been repeated several times as ascending potency. The genito-urinary tract has now functioned perfectly for the past year, blood pressure is good, and no night frequency. The vertigo returns just occasionally, the arteries are soft and compressible. His general health has improved tremendously and he is now a well man, whereas two years ago he was going down hill, and fairly rapidly at that.

Mrs. A.M. age 55 years, large and very much overweight. Four children. Varicose veins of both legs very painful. Veins in lower legs stood out like ropes. A depressed patient, cries easily and without cause. Oppression of breathing very marked in damp, cold weather. Haemorrhoids for many years, dating back to first pregnancy. *Calc Fluor* 30 was given, single dose, and was repeated in various potencies over a period of eighteen months. The varicose veins have greatly reduced in size and have never pained her since the first month of treatment. The haemorrhoids have disappeared, she is no long troubled with oppressed breathing in damp weather and looks a picture of health.

CHAPTER 15

Questions and Answers

In response to the many questions received from busy practitioners, advanced students and laity for guidance on particular points of the homoeopathic art, it is our intention to answer a cross section of these questions which we feel will be of interest to our many readers.

Q. A.C.L. writes:
Boy of five years, whose chronic remedy is *Silica*. Two weeks after a 10M dose he comes down with what appears to be a clear Phosphorus bronchitis.
1. Would you repeat the *Sil.*, and if so in what potency?
2. Or would you give *Phos.* (what potency?) — and if so would it interfere with the course of the chronic remedy. How soon after recovery from bronchitis would you repeat the *Sil*?
3. Would you simply give general care?

A. *The bronchitis is either an acute or an exacerbation of a part of the chronic brought out by the* Sil. 10M.
It is the nature of chronic disease to subside when an acute is actively present; in that case, the acute case, standing alone, should be prescribed for upon its own symptoms without fear of disturbing the chronic.
Should the bronchitis be a part of the chronic, remember that a remedy which can bring a symptom or group of symptoms to the surface usually has power to cure those symptoms without further medication, therefore it is time to watch and wait. There is another thing to be remembered and that is when any part of a chronic case is so actively present that it threatens the immediate life of the patient, it must be prescribed for even though that prescription should prolong the chronic case.
'How soon would you repeat the chronic remedy?' — *Just as soon as the chronic symptoms return and demand it.*
'Would you simply give general care?' — *Give general care and consideration at every stage of a case.*

Q. S.E.D. writes:

Girl of sixteen with hollow, fairly continuous cough (whenever she has a cough it has the hollow quality, since whooping cough five years ago); chest clear; no modalities as to time, position, air, motion or drinking. Whatever is raised must be swallowed; moderately chilly; no perspiration; slight stitching pains in both ears, worse on cough. Gave *Causticum* 1M, later *Hepar Sulph* 2c three doses at two hourly intervals. Occasional gagging but the cough persists. Please advise.

A. *The case is chronic. With that in mind take it again, then if the case is still mixed remember that when a suppressed disease (whooping cough?) is the disturbing cause in a case its nosode or remedy that was indicated at that time, if particulars can be obtained, will often turn the case into order and show the curative remedy.*

Q. D.N. writes:
How do you select the homoeopathic antidote?

A. *I select it from Hering's 'Guiding Symptoms' on the rare occasions it is needed. When your remedy fits the patient like a glove and especially if structural changes have taken place, give a fairly low potency — not above 30th, it will avoid the necessity of antidoting.*

Q. M.K.S. writes:
Mrs.— aged 45, a migraine sufferer for many years on who such apparently well indicated remedies as *Sanguinaria; Iris;* and *Psorinum* have failed to have any effect. Would you please advise on approach to this case.

A. *(1) Take the constitutional symptoms of your patient.*
(2) Take the particular symptoms of the migraine attack.
(3) Bring 1 and 2 together under the one remedy — that is your similimum. I have never failed to cure a case of migraine by adopting this method.

Q. Mrs. P.M.:
I am 55 years and quite well in myself, but my feet ache so dreadfully from walking. I am a supervisor in a large departmental store and consequently on my feet all day; my local doctor simply says 'change your job' but that is easier said than done for a woman at my time of life. Can you please help me.

A *Take Arnica 3X tablets, 1 — three times daily for one week only.*

> *A hot footbath each night of Arnica ø, one fluid drachm to the gallon of hot water after which massage in Oil of Arnica locally. This is a wonderful restorative for tired feet.*

Q. Mrs. C.H.T. writes:
I am told I have arthritis in my fingers, they feel stiff and painful and when I try to close my hand the pain in the finger joints is awful. Have tried many treatments but nothing seems to help.

A. *All rheumatic and arthritic cases should be investigated by a professional homoeopath but as from the balance of your letter I see this is not possible in your case try Caulophyllum 3X, 2 tablets 4-times daily for 7 days only; it may well palliate the pain in your fingers.*

Q. Mr. R.M. writes:
For 12 years I have suffered from piles which, although they have cleared up on occasions, I have now been advised to have them removed surgically. I am an accountant by profession and being seated most of the day the piles cause me great discomfort.

A. *I have never yet had occasion to send a patient with haemorrhoids to the surgeon. Haemorrhoids (piles) will always respond to homoeopathic treatment and I suggest you make an effort to contact a skilled homoeopath in your district who will speedily correct this disorder and avert the necessity of surgical interference.*

Q. Mrs. Mayhew, Luton, writes:
'I have been much encouraged lately with the amount of interest shown in Homoeopathy that several of us are hoping we can get sufficient to make more public meetings worth while. Converts have been won through receiving the benefit of Homoeopathy for shingles in the eye. One lady I knew fairly well was in awful pain and her eye was terribly inflamed, and after she was cured with *Rhus-tox* the doctor was amazed and told her he quite expected her to lose the eye.
She longed to tell him how she was cured, but as he didn't ask, although she told him that she had stopped taking his medicine, she felt perhaps it was better not to do so, in case she hurt his feelings. The pain and inflammation subsided in one day after three doses of *Rhus-tox* 30, so that she was able to go on holiday two days later.
Another, a friend's husband, developed shingles in face and

eyes, with severe rash; at first he thought he was affected by paint he was using but when the Dr. diagnosed shingles I was contacted at once. Again *Rhus-tox* 30 proved its worth and when he visited his doctor four days later saying he was quite fit and ready for work, all the doctor could say was 'Well you're a lucky man" — repeating this three times. When a third case was treated with the same good results — I'm wondering if we can call *Rhus-tox* almost specific for this type of trouble?'

A. *In a high percentage of simple, uncomplicated cases of Herpes Zoster (Shingles), Rhus-tox will be indicated and the 30th potency is ideal, but there are a number of cases Rhus-tox will NOT cure and a comparative study of the skin lesions of such remedies as Ran-B., Mez., Ars-alb. and Variolinum to mention those most commonly required, will enable one to speedily differentiate, and accurately select the curative remedy.*
    But, as I have said, Rhus-tox will more often be indicated than other remedies.

Q. D — writes 'I have a patient, a civil engineer age 36 years, who has responded splendidly to constitutional treatment. He was suffering from asthma, which had been with him since childhood as a result of which his general health had been greatly affected. He is out of asthma now and anti-psoric remedies have been mainly used in remoulding him constitutionally, but he still has asthma, be it mildly, whenever he is around horses or near to someone who has been recently. Can anyone give a clue to a remedy or remedies controlling this condition?'

A. *From your letter, and the classical prescribing you have applied to this patient, I am a little surprised that this allergy persists. As you will know, whan a patient has enjoyed the advantages of constitutional prescribing, these allergic states so often disappear. I would suggest the occasional dose of Pothos Foetidus 30, it may well desensitize this patient.*

Q. M.W.H. writes 'In a case of whooping cough, if you have given a partially similar remedy which has helped temporarily but the cough has returned and now you see the true similimum which you should have given in the first place, can you now give it?"

A. *Under these circumstances, by all means give the remedy at once.*

Q. Dr. — writes 'What remedies are suitable in severe auricular fibrillation?'

A. *For a case of auricular fibrillation select the homoeopathic remedy on the same basis as for any other condition, paying particular attention to the general symptoms preceeding the attack. The tendency is to pay too much attention to the outstanding pathological symptoms and thus exclude from consideration many deep remedies in which these symptoms may not have been conspicuous in the provings, for it is rare that provings are carried to such an extreme extent as to bring out this type of symptom. As an illustration of types of remedies which have a most impressive record in curing many heart disorders, and which if the symptoms agree may be indicated in cases of auricular fibrillation, compare the following: Ars-alb., Cact., Carbo-v., Crot-h., Gels., Kalm., Lach., Naja., Phos., Sep. Many more could be suggested, but bear in mind that each and every patient must be prescribed for on his or her individual idiosyncrasies. The most help comes from the remedy that covers the starting point of the trouble.*

Q. Mrs. L.A. writes: 'My doctor says I have arthritis of both my knees, they have been swollen and painful for nearly a year and apart from relieving the pain he says he cannot do much more for me. I am only forty-nine and there are so many things I would like to do. Would Homoeopathy help me?'

A. *Go to a first-class Homoeopath, and in view of the fact the condition has only been with you for a year, I would say the answer is almost certainly YES.*

Q. Dr. — writes 'Why are there not more than three chronic miasms?'

A. *Perhaps there are more than three. Possibly there are only two. This question is by no means a settled one. Hahnemann recognised three chronic miasms, namely, psora, syphilis and sycosis. It is possible that tuberculosis and other disease entities would be added to the list and still leave psora flourishing in the foreground, for psora seems to be a general dumping ground for anything and everything. Certainly it is that psora has a far deeper and wider range than its mere relation to suppressed scabies. Any and all suppression of disease manifestation is detrimental and the very antithesis of curative action.*

Q. Mr. A.O.T. writes 'Where can I find a list of the acute remedies which go well after certain deep-acting chronic remedies, viz: *Allium Cepa* after *Sulph*? Theoretically *Allium* is good as an intercurrent with *Sulph*. because it contains it. Would *Puls*. be a good intercurrent with *Kali-mur* cases on the same principle, or is it not a principle?'

A.   *Dr. Gibson Miller's little book on the 'Relationship of Remedies' is the best one that I know of.*

Q.   Dr. — writes 'A patient has been greatly benefited by *Sulph* in ascending series of single doses. The symptoms now point to *Causticum*. In 'Relationship of Remedies' I see that *Causticum* antidotes *Sulph*. Dare one give the *Causticum* following the *Sulph*, or should there be some intercurrent, and if so how do you determine it?'

A.   *When Sulph has done so much for a patient it would be a pity to antidote it. What are the Causticum symptoms? Are they produced by some new influence coming in with some acute trouble? If so, then give Causticum, it will be used up in combating the acute symptoms and will not touch the Sulph. Are the Causticum symptoms a group of symptoms that have come to the surface by the action of Sulph, in the unravelling of the case? If so, they should go under the influence of the remedy which brought them up.*

Q.   Mr. L.W.S. writes: A lady of sixty having been cured of life-long migraine headache and of severe bleeding piles by Sulph and Psorinum over a period of a year, now presents the following picture:
Cannot eat more than a few mouthfuls of solid food though takes plenty of liquid nourishment — no difficulty in swallowing, no distress after solid food, simply averse to it. Complains of indigestion characterised by empty eructations without any distension. Often wakes with it between 1 and 3 a.m. Indefinite pains in abdomen (abdomen and stool negative), not very chilly; eructations incomplete; has been very unhappy since her mother's death two years ago though rarely speaks of her sorrow; attacks of belching are eased by hot drinks. Temporary relief from *Cham 200. Kali C., Nux V., Ign* and *Sulph*. given at intervals during the last two months without relief. Can you please suggest a remedy.

A.   *Nat. Mur. stands out strong in the case as presented. It also has headaches and haemorrhoids. I wonder if it could not have covered the case in the first place.*

Q. Mr. D.P. writes: Which repertory do you think is the best for accurate prescribing?

A. *Assuming that one has a thorough knowledge of Materia Medica, which is essential for accurate remedy selection, then Professor Kent's great work is I think the easiest to use for everyday prescribing, but I use Boenninghausen's also and find it extremely useful to reconstruct a case when one has only the scantiest of information to work with, and in those chronic cases where several remedies emerge, only in shadowy outlines, from a background that is a network of chronic symptoms, even more intricately woven.*

Q. Mrs. G.M.R., age 40 years writes 'My periods worry me, they are sometimes early, sometimes a week late, at times very heavy and others very slight. Does this signify anything in particular? In myself I feel quite well.

A. *It is not possible to diagnose without seeing a patient, and whilst the condition you mention may not be difficult to correct, it does mean that you should be investigated to establish the exact nature of this irregularity, and also your constitutional state, which is possibly in some way responsible for the erratic behaviour of the menstrual periods.*

Q. Mr. and Mrs. A.P.H write: Are homoeopathic medicines in any way dangerous, do they have any side effects and what is meant by reactions one reads of in homoeopathic writings.

A. *Homoeopathic remedies are not, in any way dangerous, they do not have any unwanted and damaging side-effects, which is only one of the many advantages homoeopathy has to offer. By reaction is simply meant the patients response to treatment. In this context one could say that reaction is synonymous with response.*
Your question is more fully answered in pages 7/8.

Q. Dr. — writes 'A young woman, apparently in good health, donated a pint of blood. An hour after she reached home she fainted. This was nine months ago and she has never menstruated since. How would you approach such a case?'

A. *I would suggest a complete blood count and chest X-ray in addition to a careful check on the weight trend, urine and blood pressure. Careful inquiry should be made into the patient's eating habits and mode of life and corrections made according to indications. The possibility of a tuberculous process must be considered. A case of this kind could easily have an emotional etiology (causal factor). However, a pint of one's life blood cannot be dismissed by everyone. Such a depletion might throw a borderline case completely off balance.*

Q. J.C. writes — 'Why should a day off from work or a change in routine be so upsetting to many people?'

A. *Everyone tends to become adjusted (tolerant) to his own routine no matter what that may be. As long as one is young and well, a radical departure from the regular schedule will show little effect. With advancing years, increasing pathology, gradual decline in health and decreasing adaptability, almost any change may prove upsetting or unduly fatiguing. Warning signals of this nature must be heeded and here is where the rejuvenating influence of Homoeopathic treatment is needed to arouse the constitution and grant a new lease of life. Correct case management will help in holding the ground gained by the remedy.*

Q. Nurse — writes 'In incurable cases, how does the relief given by Homoeopathic remedies compare with that of anodynes and hypnotics as given in orthodox medicine?'

A. *The Homoeopathic remedy relieves the distressing symptoms without unfortunate side effects. The mind that is under the influence of sedation cannot be really at rest or in peace. Awful dreams, hallucinations and more or less disorientation is part of the price paid for whatever relief is obtained.*

Q. Dr. — writes 'Why has it been observed that so many patients in rural communities require Sulph. as their constitutional medicine?'

A. *It is a matter of common observation that people in rural districts have less variety in their diet than those who have easier access to the larger markets of the town dweller. Certain dietary patterns if followed too rigidly, will produce definite warping of the constitution. Less variety usually means more meat, potatoes, bread and butter, etc., and these 'good nourishing foods' tend to produce a Sulph symptomatology in the course of time. It is possible that if the individual is of the lean, stoop-shouldered philosophical type, which we associate with some Sulph patients, then the trend toward Sulph would be accelerated.*

Q. Mr. C.D.P. writes — 'After a remedy has been prescribed, how soon should evidence of its action be expected?'

A.   *In very acute conditions anywhere from a few minutes to several hours. In sub-acute cases, several hours to a day. In chronic patients anywhere from one to several days. Belladonna is often indicated in very acute throat infections and it may begin to give relief in less than five minutes. Ignatia will often quiet patients with voluble, hysterical grief and much sighing in less than ten minutes. Gelsemium is generally somewhat slower paced and may require hours to show results.*
Any remedy may act quickly in acute illness and much more slowly in chronic conditions. Sometimes it is necessary to wait a week or even ten days before attempting to evaluate the patient's reaction to a medicine. This is particularly true of the deeply chronic ambulatory case.

Q.   Lady — writes 'How important are the emotions as a cause of disease?'

A.   *In our present stage of development most people live almost entirely in their emotions. The emotional appeal is apparently the only one that really counts as the advertisers have long ago discovered. Propaganda of all kinds, whether political, religious or commercial, is directed at the emotional rather than at the rational human being. The emotions of anger and resentment are among the most deleterious in their effect and a potent cause of disease.*
Long continued deep resentment is now regarded, by some, as one of the predisposing causes of malignant disease.

Q.   Mrs. M.S. of Shenfield asks: 'As one dose of a homoeopathic remedy is the same whether one pilule or powder is given or say six pilules, or even the bottle, provided it is given in one dose at one and the same time, what is the action when diluted with water. Does each spoonful amount to the same potency, and if so what happens when a dose is diluted. Is it simply assimilated into the body more quickly?'

A.   *Individual experience, individual preference, has always entered into the method of administering a remedy, but for all practical purposes, when a potentised remedy is given in water, the water, acting as a vehicle, brings that remedy into contact with a larger surface area of nerve endings through which the remedial stimulus is conveyed.*

Q.   Mr. J.H.H. of New Zealand asks: 'I have been informed

recently that *Crataegus* given for the heart can be injurious to the liver. Do you consider this is so? The information apparently came from a pharmacopaea by Martindale.'

A. *Crataegus is a safe and gentle heart tonic and there is some evidence of beneficial action on heart muscle, but there is none, after nearly a century of homoeopathic clinical use and experience with this remedy, to suggest it is in any way deleterious to liver function.*

Q. Dr. — writes: 'Would you please define what is an intercurrent remedy, when is it called for and how should it be selected?'

A. *If one wishes to do so, a long article could be written on what is at first thought a simple question. Briefly an intercurrent remedy is one given to a patient who is under the action of a chronic constitutional remedy, for the relief of an acute miasm or for the relief of a group of severe, painful, acute symptoms; it is selected as any remedy is selected, on the totality of the acute group.*
Another example is when there seems to be lack of reaction to a well chosen remedy and on re-taking the case one can see no other remedy, and change in potency of the remedy given does not produce results; an intercurrent dose of a nosode — in line with the patients constitution or family history, even if not many of the symptoms seem to agree — has often given striking results. Often after one such deep dose the previous, apparently inactive remedy, will take hold.

Q. Mrs. C.S.M. writes: 'I am 41 and have suffered from chronic constipation since childhood, would Homoeopathy help me?'

A. *Most certainly yes, chronic constipation leads to absorption into the system of poisonous waste products, creates general debility and a host of other disorders, and nearly always has a constitutional background.*
Homoeopathic medicines, accurately selected for the patients personal requirements will do much to correct the condition.

Q. Mrs. H.S. writes: 'My daughter aged 17 years has not commenced her menstrual periods and I am so worried that she will be given drugs which may damage her constitution. Can you advise me please?'

A. *I suggest you seek the services of a professional homoeopath as the condition you mention, speedily and naturally responds to homoeopathic treatment and the patients constitutional state is always great benefited.*

Q. Mr. W.H.S. writes: 'What exactly is the difference between an acute and chronic remedy?'

A. *Some remedies act longer and deeper than others and are referred to as chronic remedies. They may be equally useful in acute conditions and any remedy may cure a chronic case but it is more generally accepted that an acute remedy is one similar to the immediate symptoms of a patient suffering from an acute illness or disease. A chronic remedy is one similar to the underlying constitutional state which was present before the acute trouble occurred and remains after it has cleared up. A patient on a chronic remedy will seldom require an acute or intercurrent medicine although one must always be vigilant on this point, but patients who have been under correct homoeopathic treatment for some time will become largely immune to acute conditions.*

Q. A regular physician interested in homoeopathy asks whether insulin, thyroid and ovarian extracts should not be given to fill the immediate physiological need caused by some underlying morbid process, and whether during their administration the chronic homoeopathic remedy may not be prescribed in the hope that it will so better the case that the insulin etc., dosage can be reduced and finally omitted.

A. *Yes, supplying deficient glandular extracts, in my opinion, does not interfere with the homoeopathic remedy. However, be sure that there is a deficiency and that you do not pass beyond it, thereby masking your case. Stay just short of the needed supply. Assist nature and compel her to build up.*

Q. Dr. — writes 'Which remedies do you find most useful in cystitis and bladder troubles generally?'

A. *I have found* Cantharis *to be the most commonly indicated remedy in acute cystitis but there are many remedies to be considered and all on their own particular indications. One of the first remedies I think of in old* chronic *cases of bladder trouble is* Uva Ursi, Pareira Brava *is another. When patients have to press down with their hands on* abdomen, *in order to empty the bladder* Mag. Mur *is often the remedy. Constant urging to urinate when standing or walking often calls for* Mag. Phos.
In old bladder cases where the patient is passing blood and ropy mucus in the urine Chimaphila *Mother Tincture should be compared and it often brings great comfort to these old cases.*

For the successful treatment of any case, it is absolutely essential, to determine accurately the cause of the patient's distress. Superficial or hurried examinations often do not find the real *root* of the trouble, which is one of the reasons why treatment prescribed on the basis of such examinations so frequently proves unsuccessful.

Successful treatment does depend upon a careful and painstaking assessment of the true nature of the patient's ill-health.

Systematic Homoeopathic treatment will do much to remove hereditary taints, constitutional weakness and tendencies to disease, and help to produce robust health and vigour in place of life-long incapacity and suffering.